'As a nurse, I have previously read bc
first one that has been a real page tu
historical figure's fascinating charac
It's a truly interesting read.'

Sonya
Clinical Nurse Specialist, University College London Hospital

'Despite living nearly two hundred years ago, Elizabeth Gaskell's life still feels relevant today. Not only did she successfully balance the pressures of a career with her duties as a wife and mother, but she also bravely stepped outside the confines of Victorian womanhood to champion the disenfranchised, and challenge social hypocrisy.

While much is known about the lives of these two women, this well-researched book brings a fresh perspective to the subject by focusing on the complex psychological effects mothers and motherhood have on women's lives. Florence and Elizabeth were deeply divided on this issue. Elizabeth believed her role as a mother was crucial to her daughters' wellbeing; Florence saw things differently, and sadly those differences were never resolved.

Finally, Naomi shows the relevance of this "grand quarrel" to our own society, where the "choice" between being a working or stay-at-home mother can be emotionally challenging, with decisions often being driven purely by economic factors. Ultimately, what this study illustrates is that being a mother is perhaps the hardest job in the world!'

Dr Diane Duffy, Chair of the Gaskell Society
and Trustee of Elizabeth Gaskell's House

'The "grand quarrel" remains as pertinent today as it was in Nightingale and Gaskell's time. Then, it was almost impossible for mothers to pursue professions outside marriage and motherhood. Today the average mother lacks the economic freedom and confidence to devote a period of time to raising her family. The crux of the argument is whether child-rearing obstructs women from achieving real societal impact, or whether the emotional and vocational role of mothering actually shapes society. Institutional childcare is a means of freeing women from the "burden of care". But what do mothers lose when they give up their role to "crèches", and more importantly, are our children's needs being met by replacing "mother"?'

Anne Fennell, Chair Mothers at Home Matter,
President European Federation Parents & Carers at Home

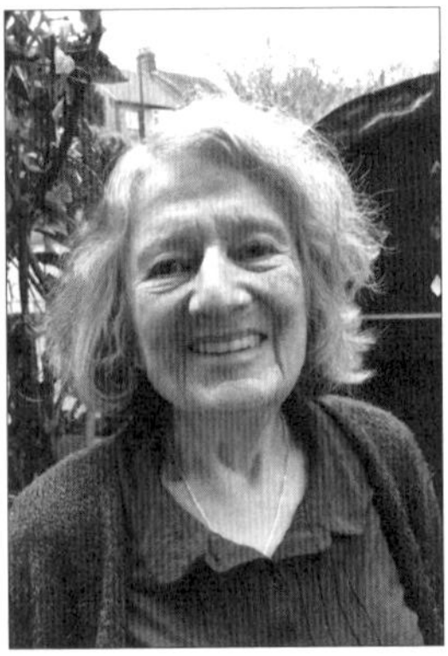

About the author

Naomi Stadlen is married to Anthony Stadlen. They have three children and three grandchildren. She has worked as an existential psychotherapist in private practice, specialising in seeing mothers and parent-couples. She has taught and supervised at the New School of Psychotherapy and Counselling. She has run Mothers Talking, a weekly discussion group on Zoom. In her spare time, Naomi enjoys Wu-style Tai Chi, quick crosswords, Jewish studies, and classical music. Further details at www.naomistadlen.com

Her books are:
What Mothers Do – especially when it looks like nothing (2004)
How Mothers Love – and how relationships are born (2011)
What Mothers Learn – without being taught (2020)
Why Grandmothers Matter (2023)
A Grand Quarrel: Elizabeth Gaskell, Florence Nightingale and mothers today (2025)

A Grand Quarrel

Elizabeth Gaskell,
Florence Nightingale
and mothers today

Naomi Stadlen

montag & martin

Photo credits:
Front cover, top left-hand medallion: portrait of Elizabeth Gaskell
Front cover, top right-hand medallion: photograph of Florence Nightingale
Front cover, main picture: sketch of Nightingale home at Lea Hurst (courtesy of British Library)
Back cover: mothers at one of Naomi Stadlen's Mothers Talking meetings (photo credit: Anita Atkinson)
Author photo page 3: Naomi Stadlen (photo credit: Anthony Stadlen)

A Grand Quarrel: Elizabeth Gaskell, Florence Nightingale and mothers today

First published by Montag & Martin Ltd 2025

ISBN 978-1-78066-820-8

Also available as ebook

Editor Susan Last

Index by Helen Bilton

British Library Cataloguing-in-Publication Data
A catalogue record for this book is available from the British Library.

Montag & Martin Limited
Unit 803 Omega Works
4 Roach Road
London E3 2PH

montagandmartin.com

Contents

Introduction

One day, I noticed a book in my local library, *Elizabeth Gaskell: A Portrait in Letters*.[1] I picked it up, and it fell open at Elizabeth Gaskell's account of her 'grand quarrel' with Florence Nightingale. It sounded like an interesting story. What did they quarrel about, and why was it 'grand'?

I started reading, and realised that here was a story that deserved to be told. The quarrel was emotional for both of them. Neither was a typical Victorian woman. They were original and bold thinkers, with ideas that are relevant today.

However, their originality has since been watered down. Today, Elizabeth is regarded mostly as a romantic novelist. That shows the most casual reading of her work. She was a profound thinker who was able to use characters in her novels to reveal many aspects of a social dilemma. Charles Dickens admired her work. Florence, too, is mostly remembered as 'the lady with the lamp'. Her later achievements are hardly recognised. She was horrified by the suffering of British soldiers that she witnessed in the Crimean War. To prevent further disease and deaths among soldiers of the British Army in India, she studied statistics, drew diagrams and became an impressive statistician. Even though she was a mere woman in 19th-century England, her command of the facts had to be respected by the most hardened Victorian Members of Parliament. Today, few of us realise how much we owe her for her insistence on hygiene routines in our homes, hospitals and the British Army.

The grand quarrel took place at Lea Hurst, Florence's family home. Elizabeth had been invited to stay there as a guest of Florence's mother. It was October 1854, and just days earlier Florence had been asked by the War Office to take a party of nurses to Turkey. They were to care for soldiers wounded in what we now call the Crimean War. The 'grand quarrel' seems to have taken place just before the appointment was officially confirmed. But

Florence must have been excited.

This might explain why she, a childless woman, explained to Elizabeth that: 'if she (Florence) had influence enough not a mother should bring up her child herself; there should be crèches for the rich as well as for the poor.' It was a bold statement. Elizabeth had four teenage daughters. Her own mother had died when she was just over a year old, so it meant a great deal to her to become a mother herself. She doesn't reveal what she replied. But it was obviously something quite strong. She described their exchange not just as a quarrel, but as a 'grand quarrel'. 'Grand' here seems to mean a major quarrel, which it surely was.

From their clear writing, it is possible to understand why both were so roused. Florence believed she was called into the service of God when she was in her teens. God, she felt, had given each woman a special gift, which meant she was capable of far more than staying at home as a wife and mother. Florence was sure that many middle-class women were as frustrated as she was. Elizabeth, however, saw motherhood as a holy undertaking, in keeping with the will of God. Being a mother was exciting, not frustrating. In other respects, they valued one another and, after the Crimean War, they continued to communicate. However, their difference was never resolved.

Why should we study a quarrel between two women in the 19th century? It's strange that the very issues they both raised presaged a split among modern women. Florence's revolutionary idea that married mothers should no longer depend on their husbands, but have independent jobs and careers, would have startled many Victorians. Yet, after two world wars, her vision has turned into ordinary reality. Women today are no longer expected to remain at home to mother their children. Many children attend crèches, child-minders and nurseries, if these are available, often as babies, while their mothers return to their paid work. This change is not seen as extraordinary. These mothers appear to be living Florence's dream.

Elizabeth's belief in motherhood, which seemed so obvious

in the 19th and early 20th centuries, is now considered reactionary. Those mothers who can afford to spend more time caring for their children are often regarded as self-indulgent, and as failing to support the workforce. Others would prefer to care for their children, especially during the early years, but haven't the funds to leave their paid work. Some define themselves as feminists because, they say, their work as mothers empowers them. But they have not been accepted by mainstream feminists (who regard paid work as the source of power), nor are they much respected by the society we live in. As one mother wrote to me: 'I have stopped work to look after my young boys, and it is amazing how counter-cultural and isolating this feels at times – I call the pram my "invisibility cloak"!'

So, in the final chapter of *A Grand Quarrel,* we shall emerge from the 19th century to explore the essential problems that mothers face today. It wasn't easy to write this, but, after raising my own children, I have facilitated a weekly discussion forum for mothers for over 34 years, and learned from it. However, the larger part of the book, chapters 1 to 9, examines not just the quarrel itself, but also the crucial issues and experiences that Florence and Elizabeth brought to it. Their writings are brilliant and provide a clear perspective on their polarised views. You may be drawn to one side more than the other. But we need both. We need Florence Nightingale *and* Elizabeth Gaskell.

Author's Note

I feel very awkward using the first names of Elizabeth Gaskell and Florence Nightingale. It seems intimate, and perhaps even disrespectful. But, because this discussion includes their families, there are several Gaskells and Nightingales, so using first names avoids confusion. Chapter 10, however, is not about their families, so I have reverted to their surnames.

Where mothers are quoted but not referenced, this is because their words come from statements made to me, either in writing or in one of my Mothers Talking discussion meetings.

I

Elizabeth Gaskell, Florence Nightingale

Chapter 1

A visit to Lea Hurst

The 'grand quarrel' took place at Lea Hurst, a beautiful stately home in the Derbyshire hills. It belonged to the Nightingale family, and Elizabeth Gaskell had been invited for a visit.

What follows is a curious story, best told through the words of both women, whenever possible. Elizabeth and Florence sound as though they wrote as they would have spoken. Their writing sounds very alive. I hope, once you get used to their 'voices', that you will get a good sense of them both.

We will start by getting to know Lea Hurst. As a reader, you may be reluctant to spend time on a mere house, and prefer to hurry on to the quarrel itself. You are free to skip chapters as you choose. But you would miss something. We are in an earlier era. The 19th-century pace of life is slower, especially in a country home. People had more time for one another and for their surroundings, more time to talk and reflect, more time to *feel*. If we jump straight to the quarrel, we will lose the slow 19th-century rhythm that will enable us to appreciate many layers of meaning.

One of Elizabeth's close friends, Susanna Winkworth, left a description of her that may help us to reach this gentler pace.

> *Though one of the most brilliant persons I ever saw, she had none of the restlessness and eagerness that spoils so much of our conversation nowadays. There was no hurry or high-pressure about her, but she seemed always surrounded by an atmosphere of ease, leisure and playful geniality, that drew out the best side of everyone who was in her company.*[1]

We are fortunate in being able to approach Lea Hurst together with a contemporary journalist. We will then arrive inside the house with Elizabeth herself. Llewellyn Hewitt was a local Victorian writer who was familiar with the Derbyshire hills. He also knew about the members of the Nightingale family who were part of the local gentry. He'd read that 'their' Florence, the younger daughter, had been sent to the Barrack Hospital at Scutari in Turkey with a party of nurses, to tend to British soldiers wounded in the Crimean War. This made sense to the journalist. He was familiar with the local stories about Florence. He recalled:

> *From her earliest years, she has had a yearning sympathy with the poor, the distressed, and the desolate; and her best energies, aided by her ample fortune, have been entirely devoted to the alleviation of the sufferings and pains of her fellow creatures.*[2]

Hewitt tried to imagine Florence's role in the Crimean War. In previous conflicts, such as the Napoleonic Wars, people in England couldn't have had much idea of what war looked like. Battlefield scenes were only painted long afterwards. Older people might have remembered their fears that Napoleon was planning to invade England, as Elizabeth had described in *Cranford*. But all that was 40 years earlier. Since then, telegraphy had been invented and newspapers had become popular. *The Times* had appointed William Howard Russell as its Special Correspondent to record the battles of the Crimean War. Russell sent back graphic descriptions of wounded, diseased and dying British soldiers. There were also war artists and, for the first time, photographs from the front. Shocked readers back in Britain could see these terrible scenes for themselves.

This made it possible for Llewellyn Hewitt to visualise Florence far away at the enormous, bleak Barrack Hospital at Scutari, tending to the soldiers:

> *at the risk of her life, and despite the scenes which she must witness, and from which most people would recoil in dread, with her whole heart awakened to that distress and pain*

> *which the poor fellows must be enduring in a hospital without organisation.*[3]

What a contrast from these battle and hospital scenes it was to enjoy a ramble through the quiet hills of Derbyshire! Hewitt wrote:

> *Lea Hurst, the seat of William Edward Nightingale, Esq.* [Florence's father], *is beautifully and romantically situated on rising ground in the midst of one of the most charming and extensive of the Derbyshire valleys, and surrounded on every side with hills and mountains, rocks and woods of majestic and gigantic proportion, and watered by the winding Derwent and its tributary streams.*[4]

He walked through the villages of Holloway, Dethick and Lea, where it was quiet enough to hear 'the musical though almost monotonous trickling and rippling of the little brook,'[5] probably a tributary of the River Derwent. He mentioned that there was now a railway line 'with its rushing fiery engines' running between the Derwent and the Old Matlock Road. At last, he reached Lea Hurst itself:

> *The Hall, erected in Elizabethan style, is most enchantingly situated on an expansive sloping lawn on the outer edge of an extensive park, and is surrounded and overhung with luxuriant trees.*[6]

It sounds peaceful. Elizabeth had been there a few months earlier and was impressed by it too. At the end of her visit, she wrote to a friend: 'It [Lea Hurst] is so lovely; so very lovely, and still, and out of the world; to say nothing of the air more pure than any I have ever yet felt.' She noticed the pure air because it must have been such a contrast to the smoky air of industrial Manchester. In 1850, the Gaskells moved to a large house on the outskirts of Manchester where Elizabeth kept poultry and grew vegetables.

But this couldn't compare with the fresh air of acres of parkland, woods, and traditional Derbyshire cottages and small villages beyond. In a letter to Parthenope, Florence's older sister, Elizabeth wrote: 'I wanted to render thanks for my happy happy pause of life at Lea-Hurst!'[7] By 'pause of life' she probably meant that she felt well cared for through the efficient management of the large house by Fanny Nightingale. She had no domestic responsibilities, but needed to be sociable at mealtimes and to finish writing her novel. Once she got home, the whole weight of domestic organisation that she had to carry would be back on her shoulders.

Fanny Nightingale, Florence's sociable mother, enjoyed inviting and hosting interesting guests. She had two daughters, and saw it as her duty to ensure that both would marry well. Their husbands should be excellent and respectable gentlemen of the Nightingale family's own class or better. By 1854, both daughters were in their early thirties and neither had married. So plenty of eligible men – cousins, friends, authors, politicians, cabinet ministers and other suitable upper-class contacts – were invited to stay at Lea Hurst or the Nightingales' larger house at Embley. Florence never did marry, and her mother might have thought her efforts had been in vain. But far from it. Those early contacts would have given Florence a very good preparation for later on, when she had to create her own networks of loyal supporters.

In 1854, Fanny invited a controversial novelist of national fame to stay. The family had met Elizabeth Gaskell through their social circle in London, much earlier, when Elizabeth had only just started publishing essays and short stories. Florence mentioned her casually in a letter dated May 1839: 'We have seen Lady Sitwell and Mrs Gaskell several times.'[8] Since then, Elizabeth had brought up a family and published three novels. Charles Dickens admired her work, and had published her stories and essays in his weekly journal *Household Words*. Now she was at work on a fourth novel, *North and South*. As a special experiment, Dickens offered to publish the entire novel as a serial, in 20 consecutive issues of *Household Words*. He was taking a risk as she hadn't finished writing it, so he didn't know how it would end. She had sent him the first part and he had already published 13 chapters. Soon he would need the rest. The plan was that she would have a quiet room at Lea Hurst where she would be undisturbed and could bring her novel to completion.

Elizabeth accepted the invitation and arrived at Lea Hurst in October 1854. However, when Fanny Nightingale invited her, she could not have predicted how crucial that October was going to be for her younger daughter, Florence. In June 1854, the British and French governments joined the Turkish side in the war against Russia. British troops had already been sent to the Crimea to counter Russian forces there. In those summer months, the Nightingale family didn't seem affected by the distant war. Life continued as usual. It was only after the Battle of the Alma in September 1854, a battle won by the British, that concerns were raised in the newspapers about the terrible injuries suffered by British soldiers.

Florence was then the superintendent of a hospital in Harley Street, London. Her reputation as a trained, competent nurse and brilliant administrator had spread. In October, she was invited by the War Office to gather and lead a team of nurses to the Barrack Hospital at Scutari (modern Üsküdar, district of Istanbul). It was an extraordinary commission and caused a national sensation. No nurse had ever been funded by the War Office to work for the British Army. And Nightingale had less than a week between learning of her appointment and setting off with her nurses. She had been assured that the hospital would have all the equipment that she would need. But she wasn't convinced, and ordered more essential supplies herself. Suddenly, peaceful Lea Hurst was in turmoil. The Nightingale family rallied round to support Florence, which meant leaving their country home for London. Elizabeth, who had only recently arrived, at Mrs Nightingale's invitation, was left behind.

We are fortunate that Elizabeth was a superb letter-writer. She must have brought a supply of her quill pens, ink and writing paper with her. 'I cannot *mend* quill pens,' she wrote, '& cannot write easily with *steel* pens.'[9] And she ran out of decent writing paper towards the end of her stay at Lea Hurst. She wrote to a friend: 'I am very much ashamed of my paper; but I am 3 miles from any kind of shop.'[10]

She had arrived at Lea Hurst a few days before the family left, and was fascinated by the house and everyone in it, especially Florence. The first letter from there to her friend Catherine Winkworth was dated 11–14 October, suggesting that it had been written in instalments with interruptions in between.

Elizabeth wasn't the only guest. There were several other people staying. 'And now I'm going to tell you bits of fun &c,' was how she introduced the other guests in her letter. 'They have had Mr Hallam, Lord Monteagle, Sir Francis Doyle & several others staying here & all the talk was about Whewell's book the Plurality of Worlds or whatever it is.'[11] From her account of their jocular discussion, Elizabeth must have been present, listening to every word. Their conversation amused her. She didn't comment that these men had a well-known female author in their midst, and that 'all the talk' could have been about her work. She recognised the typical Victorian male gathering, and was almost certainly collecting turns of phrase that she would use later in her novels.

She marvelled at the beautiful view as Hewitt had, but from a window inside Lea Hurst. What a contrast to the bustle of Manchester where she lived! Sitting in Florence Nightingale's old bedroom, she described, with her writer's precision, what she could see:

> *one low window on one side trellised over with Virginia Creeper as gorgeous as can be; and the opposite one, by which I am writing looking over such country! First a garden with stone terraces and flights of steps, and old stone columns with globes at the top of them in every direction – the plane of these terraces being perfectly gorgeous with masses of hollyhocks, dahlias, nasturtiums, geraniums, &t – Then a sloping meadow losing itself in a steep wooded – (such tints!) descent to the river Derwent, the rocks on the other side of which form the first distance & are of a red colour streaked with misty purple.*

> *Beyond interlacing hills forming three ranges of distance – the first dun brown with decaying heather, the next in some mysterious purple shadow & the last catching some pale watery sun-light. I don't know where it comes from!*[12]

Her description is so precise that an artist visited Lea Hurst one October and decided to paint the scene, partly from its present appearance and partly using her account.

And what about the rooms where she had to sit and finish her novel?

> *I am established high up, in two rooms opening one out of the other; the old nurseries, the inner one – very barely furnished – is my bedroom now; but usually Miss* [Parthenope] *N's. It is curious how simple it is compared even to that of our girls. The carpet does not cover the floor, it is far from new. The furniture is painted wood; no easy chair, no sofa, a little curtainless bed; a small* [looking] *glass not so large as mine at home. One of the windows opens out onto a battlement from which, high as Lea Hurst is, one can see the clouds careering around one; one seems on the Devil's pinnacle of the earth. It is curious to see how simply these 2 young women have been brought up.*

Florence Nightingale's room was just as bare as her sister's.

> *In the outer room – the former day nursery – Miss FN's room when she is at home every thing is as simple; now of course the bed is reconverted into a sofa, two small tables, a few empty bookshelves a drab carpet only partially covering the clean boards, and stone coloured walls – as cold in colouring as needs to be.*[13]

William Nightingale had inherited money, so the family was very wealthy. Elizabeth had four daughters and studied the two rooms with motherly eyes. It must have seemed strange to see the spartan furnishings, compared to the comfortable ones that she imagined

Parthenope and Florence could have had.

She knew what it was like to be poor. 'I have known well', she wrote in a letter to an unnamed mother, 'what it is to be both wanting money, & feeling weak in body and entirely disheartened.'[14]

She was given these two rooms because they were set apart from the rest of the household, and would enable her, urged by an anxious Dickens, to write undisturbed. Fanny Nightingale was a thoughtful hostess. Elizabeth continued:

> *It is getting dark. I am to have my tea, up in my turret – at 6. – And after that I shall lock my outer door & write. I am stocked with coals, and have candles up here; for I am a quarter of a mile of staircase & odd intricate passage way from everyone else in the house. Could solitude be more complete! The house is in a wild park, along which I hardly yet know my way so as to get to the different gates.*[15]

Knowing that she was stocked with enough coal to warm her while writing on chilly October evenings must have seemed luxurious. Elizabeth had grown up with her Aunt Lumb in Knutsford, a small town, like the one she described in her second novel, *Cranford*. In Cranford, the narrator explained, the women practised 'elegant economy'. Years later, Elizabeth's daughters visited Knutsford. They saw it more critically and concluded: 'They lived in gt poverty in Knutsford.'[16]

As for candles, they too were a feature in *Cranford*. The narrator of the novel described how candles

> *were usually brought in with tea; but we only burnt one at a time. As we lived in constant preparation for a friend who might come any evening (but who never did), it required some contrivance to keep our two candles of the same length, ready to be lighted as if we burnt two always.*

Then follows a telling detail:

> *The candles took it in turns; and, whatever we might be talking about or doing, Miss Matty's eyes were habitually fixed upon the candle, ready to jump up and extinguish it and light the other before they had become too uneven in length to be restored to equality in the course of the evening.*[17]

Was this a memory of her childhood in Knutsford with her Aunt Lumb, or a friend? If so, the plentiful supply of candles at Lea Hurst must have delighted her. 'Will you tell Mrs Nightingale,' she wrote to Parthenope, 'that I am so comfortable and cosy, and undisturbed up here? and thank her for all her kindness.' The letter is dated 17 October 1854, when the Nightingale family rushed to London. It sounds as if there hadn't been time for Gaskell to hurry down 'the quarter of a mile of staircase' to thank her hosts in person.

A day or two earlier, Elizabeth had confided to her oldest daughter, Marianne:

> *Mr and Mrs and Miss* [Parthenope] *N leave here tomorrow. I shall feel very queer in this large house by myself. At first the servants will be here, packing up things; but after that the gardener & his wife come into the house; they will live in one part, far far away, & I have all the rest of the large place to myself.*[18]

She was warm-hearted and sociable. Parthenope seems to have taken her on walks around the neighbourhood, and Elizabeth, despite being under pressure to keep writing, found time to visit some of the local cottages and enjoy talking to everyone there.

Besides, she wasn't completely alone. Provided she kept her door open, 'One companion I have got – an *owl*. Miss Florence N. picked it up – thrown out of the nest in the Parthenon – nursed the little round puff-ball...& here he is, a regular intelligent mischievous pet.'[19]

Elizabeth and Florence shared a sensitive compassion for creatures, especially helpless ones. As it turned out, Florence had saved the owl's life when it was an owlet. Now, four years later, Elizabeth would try to revive the owl after it had died.

Chapter 2

Parthenope: 'Athena, an owlet from the Parthenon'

From a very young age, Florence Nightingale felt compassion for the sick and vulnerable. Neither Nightingale sister would bear children. At the time of Elizabeth's visit, both were in their thirties, at an age when a woman would be expected to have married and borne at least one child. However, Parthenope and Florence were still hosting and going to parties, and to other social engagements, as eligible women.

Four years before the Crimean War, Florence brought Athena the owl into their lives. Athena seems to have entered their family as if she were a surrogate wilful child, a 'child' the sisters could look after together. She brought out tender motherly feelings in both of them. Parthenope, an excellent artist, sketched a number of drawings of Athena. When Florence fell ill at Scutari in 1855, and spent time convalescing, Parthenope wanted to comfort her. She used her drawings to illustrate a brief history of the 'Life and Death of ATHENA an owlet from the Parthenon'. She penned the text in a beautiful clear hand. Most of this chapter is based on her attractive work.[1]

Florence had visited Athens in the spring of 1850. She was passing under the walls of the Acropolis when she noticed a group of children tormenting something. She went over to look and saw it was a baby owl that must have fallen out of its nest. She offered the children some coins to leave the owlet alone, picked up the tiny bird, and took care of her. She managed so well that she kept Athena alive and happy for the remainder of her tour to Italy, Vienna and Berlin. Parthenope describes how, one quiet autumn evening, her sister returned to Lea Hurst, surprising herself and their mother by stepping through the drawing-room window. Florence talked to them both for half an hour before putting her hand into her pocket and pulling out a little bag. Parthenope recalled: 'Athena's head stuck out, the bag being tied about her neck; she seemed, however, very happy and very warm. When set at liberty she began while sitting on the table, to curtsey and bow with the greatest urbanity.'

So Athena entered the Nightingale family. She intrigued an elderly great aunt, Miss Evans, sister of the grandmother on their father's side. Miss Evans, Parthenope remembered, 'looked upon Athena as her great great niece,' and would ask after her welfare with solicitous dignity.

Athena sounds less like a pet and more like the youngest member of the family. 'She objected extremely to being laughed at,' observes Parthenope. The family studied her cries and identified five different sounds. 'A bark when she was naughty, a crow when she was proud, a little purr (a sort of twee twee) when she was pleased, a grumble when she was cross & a hoot when she was melancholy.' This superb level of observation sounds very similar to the way Elizabeth learned to understand her baby daughter, as we shall see in the next chapter.

Elizabeth was told the story of Athena's rescue and had already met her. But, unfortunately, when the family rushed to London to join Florence and help her prepare for her expedition to Scutari, Athena was accidentally locked in a cold room, and there she died. Elizabeth had the unenviable task of breaking the news to the family. She wrote to Parthenope next day:

> *The poor poor little Owl is dead. Last night about five in came Mrs Watson almost in tears. 'Oh dear, Mrs Gaskell whatever shall we do?' (She had it in her hands.) 'It was quite well at dinner time hopping about my room; and just now I found it on its back stiff and cold.' I took it in my hands. I fancied I could just feel a fluttering, and I held it between my warm hands near the fire. But it was but a fancy; it must have died in some fit, I imagine.*[2]

The helpless little owl brought out a similar compassion and warm tenderness for helpless animals in Elizabeth to that of Florence. Many women would have flinched from holding a dead owl, but Elizabeth held it until she was sure that she could not revive it. Since then, the owl has been stuffed, and is now at the Nightingale Museum in London.

Florence was heartbroken. Athena had lived with them for four years. Even while they were in Germany, while Florence stayed at Kaiserswerth, Parthenope had taken care of Athena for her. She was calm as she prepared for the voyage to Scutari, but wept when Athena's body was brought to her in London. 'Poor little beastie,' she said, 'it was odd how much I loved you!'.

Months later, on 5 March 1855, during a beautiful early spring evening, Florence took a walk along a cliff near Scutari. She wrote to her family in great excitement:

> *I saw Athena last night. She came to see me. I was walking home late from the Gen'l Hosp'l round the cliff, my favourite way, & looking, I really believe for the first time, at the view – the sea glassy calm & of the purest sapphire blue – the sky one dark deep blue – ...when Athena came along the cliff quite to my feet, rose upon her tiptoes, bowed several times, made her long melancholy cry, & fled away – like the shade of Ajax. I assure you, my tears followed her.*[3]

Chapter 3

Gaskell: 'I feel myself so unknowing'

We've looked at Lea Hurst where the quarrel took place, but we need to understand more about the two protagonists. Their quarrel was about the role of women and mothers. Elizabeth and Florence started from completely different life experiences. Elizabeth missed the mother that she didn't have, while Florence was thwarted by the disapproval of a mother as strong-willed as herself. Both women testify to the importance of their mothers. And yet, despite the accession of Queen Victoria in 1837, their era was dominated by the power of men.

There are two chapters on Elizabeth and two on Florence, which will take you up to the quarrel. Chapter 7 leads to the quarrel itself, and I hope by then you will have an intimate understanding of the two women and both sides of the argument.

Florence was the more dramatic writer of the two. But Elizabeth, though quieter, had perceptive insights.

We'll start with some basic facts of Elizabeth's life.

She was sufficiently 19th-century to say nothing about her seven births. And yet, they must have been powerful experiences. Giving birth can feel overwhelming, and shake a woman to her core. God, or life-spirit, or a force beyond herself had enabled a new person to grow inside her, nurtured but not created by her. Was it painful, especially the first time, and was she afraid? She was a strong woman, but did she tear in giving birth? Her silence is a lost opportunity.

Once each of her babies was born from the safety of her body, and Elizabeth could see the new child for the first time, how did she feel? She and her husband would have said prayers of thanksgiving.

'Blessed,' was the word Elizabeth frequently used about each child. Each baby surely felt like a gift from the divine.

She had been brought up by her mother's oldest sister. Elizabeth records no early memories of her own mother. Besides, she was her mother's eighth child. Her mother must by then have been experienced. Elizabeth had to think how to bring up her first baby.

Elizabeth's very first baby was stillborn. It must have been a tremendous shock, even at that time, for a woman to carry a baby for nine months who did not survive. Yet she saw it as an opportunity for love. She was only 22. She grieved for her child's suffering, more than her own, and believed that her child was now safe in heaven, and that 'thou, my child, from thy bright heaven see how well I keep my faithful vow to [remember] thee.'[1]

When Elizabeth became a mother of a living child, she wrote: 'I feel myself so unknowing.' Her sense of unknowing isn't surprising because she was very young when her own mother died. She wondered if she, too, would die young. So she kept a diary to be given to her first surviving daughter. She wanted to record what she was discovering, so that her daughter wouldn't have to learn about mothering entirely on her own, as she herself had.

Elizabeth recognised the importance of her role. It's often women who have been orphaned young who can tell us, much more clearly than those of us who have grown up with our mothers, what they have missed. To her, the value of mothers was obvious. Fortunately, she was an observant writer. Her observations are relevant today because the essentials of mothering seem eternal, and she has recorded many of them.

Elizabeth's mother, Elizabeth Holland Stevenson, bore about eight children in 13 years. Only two survived: the firstborn John and the youngest, Elizabeth Cleghorn Stevenson. A cryptic note is added by the historian John Chapple in Appendix A to the list of her children: '?Six children, d young.'[2] The reason we know so little about Elizabeth's siblings is because, unfortunately, little information is available about Elizabeth's mother. Jenny Uglow, Elizabeth's biographer, pointed out that this was typical:

> *About* [William Stevenson's] *first wife there is silence. As so often – as with Charlotte Brontë, George Eliot, Elizabeth Barrett Browning – it is her father who dominates accounts of Gaskell's parents. We know about William, but have to speculate about her mother, Elizabeth.*[3]

Elizabeth Gaskell, in her turn, bore seven children in 13 years, in a similar way to her mother. The first was a stillborn daughter, then Marianne and Meta who both survived, a boy who died as a baby,[4] Florence who survived, Willie who died at nine months of scarlet fever, and Julia who survived.[5] Readers of Elizabeth's novels complain that so many of the characters die. But evidently this was her experience.

Elizabeth was born on 29 September 1810. Her mother died on 29 October 1811 at the age of 40. Her little daughter was just 13 months old. Did someone tell her that her mother had died? Or was she, as children sometimes were, taken to see the deceased body of her mother? She seems to have had no memory of that time, as if it had been too painful to recall.

And how much does the early death of a mother affect her child? It usually meant that the child had to be cared for by relatives. Families tended to be large, and early maternal deaths were more common then, so perhaps the whole pattern seemed normal.

Jane Austen, whom Elizabeth much admired, introduced her novel *Emma* with the brief observation that Emma Woodhouse had grown up with very little to distress her. 'Her mother had died too long ago for her to have more than an indistinct remembrance of her caresses...'[6] This seems a reasonable assumption by a writer who hadn't herself experienced the early loss of her mother. Mrs Austen, after all, would outlive her younger daughter by 10 years. However, Jane's father, the Revd George Austen, and his two sisters had been orphaned as children. Early deaths were quite common, but perhaps he and his sisters didn't talk openly about any feelings of loss they might have had. So his daughter Jane might have had little information to guide her.

William Wordsworth, almost an exact contemporary of Jane's older brother Henry, was orphaned at seven years old. He was in no doubt that the early loss of a mother mattered. In *The Prelude*, he wrote about an infant's memories of his mother. Wordsworth did not own these memories as his – but how else would he have known about them?

> *Blest the infant Babe,*
> *(For with my best conjectures I would trace*
> *The progress of our being) blest the Babe,*
> *Nursed in his Mother's arms, the Babe who sleeps*
> *Upon his Mother's breast; who, when his soul*
> *Claims manifest kindred with an earthly soul,*
> *Doth gather passion from his Mother's eye!*[7]

Here, at last, from a great poet, we get a wonderful sense of a baby's experience. Surely Wordsworth wasn't the only child to enjoy these powerful sensations of lying in his mother's arms and gazing up at her face. Just as the mother gazed passionately down at her beloved child, so her child, gazing up, sensed the strength of her passion in his own soul. Elizabeth mentions that she read Wordsworth. There's a record that Charlotte Brontë asked the publisher George Smith to lend Elizabeth a copy of *The Prelude*. But if she read, presumably, this first version of *The Prelude*, and if those lines resonated with her, she didn't mention it.

She records a happy childhood. She was brought up by her mother's older sister Hannah (Aunt Lumb), whom she loved. She spent a lot of time in the company of the Hollands, her mother's large, warm-hearted family. She doesn't seem to have acknowledged much about missing her mother, apart from the odd reference in which she described herself thus: 'Though a Londoner by birth, I was early motherless...'[8] However, she revealed the strength of her feelings in a letter written on 13 February 1849, when she was 38, in reply to one George Hope:

> *acknowledging your kindness in sending me my dear mother's letters, the only relics of her that I have, and of more value to me than I can express, for I have so often longed for some little thing that had once been hers or touched by her. I think no one but one so unfortunate as to be early motherless can enter into the craving one has after the lost mother... Those who come to me with a remembrance of them* [her parents] *as an introduction seem to have a holy claim on my regard.*[9]

The words '...touched by her' describe a child's desperate need for a physical connection. This sounds closer to Wordsworth than to the brief sentence introducing Emma Woodhouse. In Elizabeth's last novel, *Wives and Daughters*, she explained succinctly how a fictional child felt at the early loss of her mother. Like Austen's Emma Woodhouse, Elizabeth's Molly Gibson had lost her mother at a young age and, again like Emma, could hardly remember her. But unlike Emma, Molly's life was changed by her loss. In half a sentence, Elizabeth shows the effect it can have. 'Poor child! it is true that she had lost her mother, which was a jar to the whole tenour [sic] of her life'.[10] Perhaps the loss of her mother explains why Elizabeth wrote novels so imbued with sadness. Many of her heroines (including Mary Barton, Ruth, Margaret Hale, Sylvia Robson, and Molly Gibson) cry a great deal.

Both before and after she became a mother herself, it's very interesting to notice that the men in Elizabeth's life – her father, brother, husband, and, as we shall see in the next chapter, Charles Dickens – all encouraged her to write.

Elizabeth's father remarried and continued to live in London. He had two more children, and tried to support his family by writing articles, pamphlets and books. He was grateful to his wife's oldest sister, Hannah Lumb, for offering to adopt his daughter. Elizabeth occasionally visited him in London, but they were unhappy times as her step-mother didn't welcome her. In the one letter by him to Elizabeth, he urged her: 'If you should go into Wales, I expect you will keep a regular journal of what you see and remember.'[11] Did he notice that she showed signs of being a capable writer? In other ways, he was basically a busy and absent father. He died in March 1829 when she was 18.

Elizabeth's only living brother, John, born on 27 November 1798, also hoped to become a professional writer. He eventually became a seaman, and at first wrote letters to his young sister. He described life on board ship, and gave her accounts of some of the countries he had visited, including India. He begged her to write him long letters about Knutsford, the town where she lived with Aunt Lumb. He also praised her 'as both your writing and your cousin's is far superior to that of many girls of your age.'[12]

It is surely autobiographical in Elizabeth's novel *North and South* when she describes 'sea-stained letters,' from a fictional sailor brother, 'with the peculiar fragrance which ocean letters have.'[13] What happened to him? 'In fact, nobody knows what happened to John,' wrote the historian John Chapple.[14] With no definite news, how could she not miss him and long to see him again? In her fiction, there is often a brother who returns from abroad.

Elizabeth married William Gaskell on 30 August 1832, when she was 21. In 1828 he had been appointed a junior minister at the Cross Street Chapel in Manchester, and continued there until he died in 1884. He was a serious, academic man. He composed the sermons that he preached, and also, as a professor of English history and literature at Manchester New College, taught and prepared lessons. He was in a good position to appreciate Elizabeth's growing ability to write.

One way in which he would be a great help to her would be the many studies he made of Lancashire dialects. She wrote proudly to a friend:

> *My husband has lately been giving four lectures to the very poorest of the weavers in the very poorest district of Manchester, Miles Platting on 'The Poets and Poetry of Humble Life'. You cannot think how well they have been attended, or how interested people have seemed. And the day before yesterday two deputations of*

> *respectable-looking men waited on him to ask him to repeat those lectures in two different parts of the town.*[15]

William Gaskell realised that weavers might be poor, but they were not without culture. So Elizabeth was able to use some of the poems and the relevant Lancashire dialect words in her first novel, *Mary Barton*.

William wasn't wealthy and, once he was married, he was entitled to his wife's property and income. A married couple was regarded as one person before the Women's Property Acts (1870 and 1882), so what was hers became his. She didn't have any property or income when they married but eventually, very unlike a typical 19th-century wife, she earned more than he did. As a woman, she was prohibited from opening a bank account in her own name, so all she earned from her writing was paid into her husband's account and became his property. But William wasn't a typical 19th-century husband either. He encouraged her to write for publication, checked her spelling, and meticulously proof-read her work. He helped her understand her writing contracts and, scrupulous as he was, made sure she received every payment. When her children were older, she began publishing novels as well as short stories in *Household Words* and *The Cornhill Magazine.* Several of her novels were translated into French and German, and republished in America. She earned modest sums at first, but these increased with her popularity. For *Wives and Daughters* her publisher paid her a cash advance of £2,000.[16]

The next section is a study of *My Diary*. It may be too detailed for a reader impatient to get to the quarrel, but I know of no other maternal diary like it. Jenny Uglow gives a fine account of it, but comments that Elizabeth's 'fascinated absorption [in her baby] is that of all parents.'[17] Perhaps, but 'all parents' haven't made the brilliant observations that Gaskell did.

My Diary was one of Elizabeth's first pieces of serious writing before she began writing professionally. It was a private and confessional work, never intended for publication. She wrote it for her first daughter, Marianne, when she was older. Elizabeth began it in March 1835 when Marianne was nearly six months old. So there is a 'silence' over those first six months. Either Elizabeth was too busy to start a diary or, very likely, since she had lost her mother and given birth to a stillborn child, life might have seemed precarious, and she wanted to be sure that Marianne was viable first.

Elizabeth unveils an unusual picture of early mothering. She makes it obvious that it is not a matter of getting through daily chores for the baby. It's an awesome responsibility of weighing up choices, and considering their long-term consequences. After all, motherhood is a huge enterprise. No individual mother can do everything possible, let alone have time to write about it. There are areas that Elizabeth has not covered. However, just a few extracts from her diary reveal how many important issues she has brought to light.

She was very unsure of herself, and anxious to make the right decisions for Marianne. She wrote from the perspective of a practising Christian, and there's a risk that this may alienate modern readers. But a religious vocabulary can connect us to some of our most profound feelings. Elizabeth expresses her wonder at her child and her fear that she would be an inadequate mother. 'But oh Lord I pray thee to lead me right (if it be thy will) and to preserve in me the same strong feeling of my responsibility which I now feel,' she wrote.[18] Mothers today, facing the vulnerability of their newborns, express similar anxiety about making good decisions, but in secular language.

It's precisely because she felt so responsible and was so self-questioning that *My Diary* can be understood by many people today. A few of Elizabeth's dilemmas were specifically 19th-century ones, but most are universal. I have discussed some of them with groups of experienced mothers. Although Elizabeth wrote so long ago, mothers today can relate to her uncertainties. They have explored similar questions themselves.

In 1923, long after her death, 50 copies were privately published.

About 70 years later, I read one of these in the British Library and was so impressed that I made photocopies for a class of adult psychology students I was teaching. To my surprise, they came back the following week and reported: 'It didn't grab my attention.' 'She's not *saying* anything.'

That's a good example of how easily genuine mothering goes unnoticed. Many people can see mothers in action, but are completely unaware of how much sheer concern and intelligence precedes their visible actions. Here, we shall try to do justice to *My Diary*. I know of no other document like it.

My Diary has been republished as *Private Voices,* so Elizabeth's intimate reflections are now available to the reading public. The book includes a second 'private voice': a journal written by one of Elizabeth's many cousins-in-law, Sophia Holland. She too kept a diary at around the same time, when her children were young. Sophia's entries are often in note form, anecdotes jotted down in spare moments. Elizabeth's are much longer, filled with observations, questions and prayers. She blamed herself for writing so rarely. But, when she did, she needed time to develop her thoughts.

Comparing the two diaries is revealing. Both mothers were Unitarian. This meant that they didn't subscribe to the mainstream Christian concept that children were born in original sin and required the ceremony of baptism to erase it. (Baptism didn't always occur soon after birth. Jane Austen, for example, was born in December, during an exceptionally cold winter, and it was early April before she could be baptised.) Both mothers wrote about their children with love and respect. Sophia recorded what her children did, whereas Elizabeth's entries show how aware she was of being responsible for Marianne's development. Like Sophia, she noted anecdotes, but she also tried to see daily life from Marianne's perspective and understand her daughter's reasons for what she did. Her writing is sensitive and honest, and several of her entries sound as though she wrote them in tears.

After Elizabeth's mother died when she was 13 months old,

she was brought up by her mother's oldest sister, Aunt Hannah Lumb. But an aunt is not a mother, and besides, she hadn't acted as mother to Elizabeth during those influential early months. We don't know what decisions Elizabeth's mother had made during those first 13 months. In any case, now that Marianne was born, Elizabeth was alarmed at her own ignorance. Not quite 24 years old herself, she was aware that she would have to make decisions on how to bring up her child which would have long-term consequences. But she didn't know what the consequences would be.

About five months later, Elizabeth used her diary to express a conviction that was to become an issue in her quarrel with Florence Nightingale. Marianne was now 10 months old, and Elizabeth had made a number of decisions on how to bring her up. But she still felt anxious and bewildered.

> *How all a woman's life, at least so it seems to me now, ought to have a reference to the period when she will be fulfilling some of her greatest & highest duties, that of a mother. I feel myself so unknowing, so doubtful about many things in her intellectual & moral treatments already, and what shall I be when she grows older & asks those puzzling questions that children do?*[19]

Most women in the 19th century became mothers. There was limited access to contraception, and little else open to them. But not everyone took it as seriously as Elizabeth. Preparation tended to be informal. Often a girl was asked to look after her younger sibling or a cousin's or aunt's baby (as Florence Nightingale was), or she simply watched her mother. It's reassuring to discover that Elizabeth, for all her inexperience and doubts, brought up four daughters to womanhood who loved her and one another. There was none of the tension that can be found in, for example, the Nightingale family. Their 'grand quarrel' arose because Florence, as we shall see, came from a different kind of mothering history.

With the responsibilities of motherhood came a dread of the

mother dying. Although she was only 24, this fear was often in Elizabeth's thoughts. It was understandable. Both her parents had died relatively young. Her diary begins:

> *To my dear little Marianne I shall 'dedicate' this book, which, if I should not live to give it her myself, will I trust be reserved for her as a token of her mother's love and extreme anxiety in the formation of her little daughter's character.*[20]

Although modern life is safer, many mothers today shyly confess to having similar fears of dying. These fears seem to express their awareness of their unique responsibilities as mothers. It's possible that mothers everywhere and at all times have silently experienced this fear.

Gaskell was also fearful that her baby daughter would die. We should remind ourselves that Marianne was, then, her only surviving child. During her daughter's first year, she recorded in her diary:

> *She was very very ill, and I was very much afraid we should have lost her. I did so try to be resigned; but I cannot tell how I sickened at my heart, at the thought of seeing her no more.*[21]

When Marianne was ill, Elizabeth was conflicted. She did all she could for Marianne. She resorted to simple homely remedies, and consulted her local doctor. But she reproached herself more than once for being *desperate* for her daughter to survive. She believed that she ought to submit herself to the will of God as a faithful Christian and wife of a Unitarian minister. When she wrote: 'I did so try to be resigned,' she meant that she thought she should be prepared to accept whatever fate God decided for her child. This makes a significant contrast with Florence Nightingale. She, too, was a committed Christian, but she was in no doubt that God wanted a sick child to be nursed back to health. One reason that Elizabeth was to admire Florence when she visited Lea Hurst, 20 years later, might well have been because Florence wasn't resigned to letting a child die. She had by then taught herself how to nurse. In her family, she was the person that ill members asked for, because she knew how to look after patients, who survived because of her care.

Then as now, even with good nursing, some babies don't survive. Many mothers maintain one-sided 'conversations' with these 'angel' children, and Elizabeth did too. Her first daughter was stillborn. She often visited her grave, and, on the third anniversary, when Marianne was nearly two, Elizabeth wrote a sonnet, 'On Visiting the Grave of my Stillborn Little Girl':

> *I made a vow within my soul, O child,*
> *When thou wert laid beside my weary heart*
> *With marks of Death on very tender part,*
> *That, if in time a living infant smiled,...*
> *Thee have I not forgot, my firstborn, ...*[22]

She had addressed her first daughter as 'thou'. Ninety years later, the Jewish existential philosopher Martin Buber published his *Ich und Du* (translated as *I and Thou* or *I and You*), in which he maintained that babies are ready to relate to a 'thou' from the start of their lives. Interesting that, even though her first daughter didn't survive, Elizabeth seemed to sense intuitively that she could relate to her daughter as 'thou'.

Her second daughter was her first venture into mothering. Now we hear her speaking directly to Marianne, writing to her as 'you'.

> *And you too, my dearest little girl, if, when you read this, you trace back any evil or unhappy feeling to my mismanagement in your childhood, forgive me, love!*[23]

This plea to her daughter is revealing. Elizabeth seems to have started with a wonderful ability to see how two people could think differently. So she envisaged a time when Marianne might disagree with some of her mother's decisions. Though Marianne was not quite six months old, Elizabeth allowed the possibility that they might not think alike.

From the start, she saw her daughter as an individual person. It might seem obvious, and yet some mothers have found it confusing that their babies, who emerged from within their own bodies, may nevertheless differ from themselves.

Many mothers are filled with wonder at the miracle of giving birth to beautiful young children, and experience a powerful desire to protect their evident goodness. Elizabeth felt this strongly. It's much easier to express using religious terms such as 'sacred' and 'holy' or Wordsworth's 'soul'. Many mothers today experience these feelings, but find it difficult to acknowledge them, as they are uncomfortable with religious-sounding terms.[24]

Elizabeth experienced her child as a blessing from God, and therefore sacred and holy. Her diary records several examples. She observed that, at 11 months, Marianne would notice the variety of moods in the expressions of the faces of those around her. 'If we could consider a child properly,' Elizabeth wrote, 'what a beautiful safe-guard from evil would it's [sic] presence be.'[25] And: 'We had an instance lately when *some one*, in anger did what was decidedly wrong in her [Marianne's] presence, without considering how holy that little creature made the place.'[26] Elizabeth must often have heard that every person is holy, in reading of the Scriptures and during her husband's sermons in chapel on Sundays. But it was surely completely different from the passion of holding a beloved child in her arms.

Marianne sounds strong-willed, even as a baby, and this was surely because Elizabeth loved her as she was, and allowed her to be expressive.

> *I will try to describe her mentally. I should call her remarkably good tempered... She is also very firm in her own little way occasionally; what I suppose is obstinacy really, only that is so hard a word to apply to one so dear. But in general she is so good*

> *that I feel as if I could hardly be sufficiently thankful, that the materials put into my hands are so excellent, and beautiful. And yet it seems to increase the responsibility.*[27]

Despite so much anxiety, Elizabeth was enchanted by her daughter and eager to describe some of the details that she had observed in those first six months.

> *Marianne is now becoming every day more and more interesting. She looks at and tries to take hold of everything. She has pretty good ideas of distance and does not try to catch sunbeams now, as she did two months ago.*[28]

How did Elizabeth know that her daughter had been trying to catch sunbeams? She must have watched for some time, puzzled by what Marianne was doing. At four months, babies haven't yet developed complete control of their limbs. Many mothers may have seen their babies waving their arms in the air, but assumed they were only exercising their limbs. And how did Elizabeth realise that Marianne had learned, at six months, that the sunbeams were too distant? This is a unique observation. Babies were sometimes regarded as irrational or, at best, led by their emotions. But Elizabeth realised that Marianne could *think*. Pre-verbal babies teach themselves about perspective, solid objects, facial expressions, and much more, before they can stand and walk. Because Elizabeth herself was so intelligent, she recognised Marianne as a fellow rational being.

This short diary entry shows Elizabeth's ability to notice details that other people might brush aside as insignificant. For Elizabeth, detailed observations were revealing. Writing about Charlotte Brontë, 20 years later, she noted that the Brontë sisters were not fond of children, and that 'The hieroglyphics of childhood were an unknown language to them.'[29] Elizabeth chose the unusual image of 'hieroglyphics' with care. She seems to mean that the pre-verbal 'language' of childhood needs to be translated or decoded in order to be understood. Without the work to understand, the child's signals will seem a mystery, as were ancient Egyptian hieroglyphics for centuries before the discovery of the Rosetta Stone. *My Diary* is filled with examples of how much Elizabeth was learning about the language of childhood. Unlike the Brontë sisters, she was fond of children, and was learning about Marianne through the warmth of her love.

This learning seems to have been mutual. Elizabeth was fascinated to notice how much Marianne was studying herself and her husband. Not yet six months old, she seemed determined to take part in their adult conversation.

> *She catches the expression of a countenance to which she is accustomed directly, when we* [Elizabeth and her husband, William] *laugh, she laughs; and when I look attentive to William's reading, it is quite ridiculous to see her little face of gravity and earnestness as if she understood every word.*[30]

From this, we can see that even while Elizabeth looked 'attentive to William's reading', she still managed to notice what her daughter was doing. She found that Marianne would only copy the facial expressions of people she knew. She couldn't yet 'read' the faces of everyone, so perhaps this is why she was 'staring at strangers' as Elizabeth noticed. By copying her parents, she must have been teaching herself about different modes of adult communication, from shared jokes to shared serious ideas. Elizabeth was impressed, and thought it was important enough to record in her diary.

She mentioned something similar when Marianne was 15 months old. 'I am sometimes surprised to find how she understands, & tries to understand what we say amongst ourselves.'[31] Again, even when she and William or another adult were talking among themselves, Elizabeth managed to keep an eye on her daughter, whose expression showed that she was listening and doing her best to understand.

Marianne seemed in a hurry to speak. 'She will talk before she can walk,' Elizabeth predicted.[32] She made odd noises which,

Elizabeth thought, sounded like talking. What could Marianne be thinking? 'I wish we could know what is passing in her little mind,' she wrote.[33] The philosopher John Locke, nearly 150 years earlier, believed we were born with a mind that was empty, a *tabula rasa*. 'If we attentively consider new-born children,' he wrote, in itself a very unusual suggestion, 'ideas come into their minds; and... they get no more, nor other, than what experience, and observation of things, that come their way, furnish them with.'[34] This seems a reasonable guess, though babies may have already started forming ideas before they are born. Even after birth it's difficult to be sure what ideas they have. Elizabeth certainly 'listened attentively'. Yet she was right to conclude that while she would *like* to know what Marianne was thinking, she didn't. This again is important. Elizabeth was an unusual mother. It can be tempting to attribute ideas to a baby, but Elizabeth was careful not to, if she didn't have some evidence that her baby had those ideas.

Elizabeth enjoyed watching to see what interested Marianne. She often sounds as though she made decisions for her daughter spontaneously, working her reasons out later and recording them in *My Diary*. For example:

> *I try always to let her look at anything that attracts her notice as long as she will, and when I see her looking very intently at anything, I take her to it, and let her exercise all her senses upon it – even to tasting if I am sure it will do her no harm. My object is to give her a habit of fixing her attention.*[35]

'Even to tasting it' – at six months, a baby's tongue is still the most accurate sense for exploring an object. Elizabeth must have recognised this. And how did she know when something had attracted Marianne's attention? How could she be sure what particular object it was? She and Marianne must have been building up some useful pre-verbal signals to communicate with one another.

Another decision Elizabeth made was:

> *She goes to bed awake; another practice I began early... Once or twice we have had grand cryings, which have been very very distressing to me; but when I have convinced myself that she is not in pain, is perfectly well, and that she is only wanting to be taken up I have been quite firm, though I have sometimes cried almost as much as she has.*[36]

Elizabeth says she never left the room before Marianne was asleep. She was determined that Marianne should learn that she was consistent, even if her method made them both cry.

At the start of her diary, we saw that Elizabeth mentioned her 'extreme anxiety in the formation of her little daughter's character'. Mothers today often describe exactly that level of anxiety. She and they complain that, when they have to make difficult decisions, they consult parenting 'experts' for some sensible advice, only to find that – then as now – these experts contradict one another.

> *Crying has been a great difficulty for me. Books do so differ. One says: 'Do not let them have anything they cry for,' another (Mme Neckar de Saussure, sur L'Education Progressive, the nicest book I have read on the subject) says 'les larmes des enfans* [sic] *sont si amères, la calme parfait de l'âme leur est si necessaire* [sic] *qu'il faut surtout épargner les larmes.'*[37]*...if it* [the child] *is to have the object for which it is crying I would give it, directly, giving up any little occupation or purpose of my own, rather than try its patience unnecessarily. But if it is improper for it to obtain the object, I think it right to with-hold it steadily, however much the little creature may cry.*[38]

This sounds a clear rule. But unlike the rule of putting her daughter down awake, this one involved two possibilities: either Marianne would be given the object or it would be withheld from her. Elizabeth was being consistent, but her logic was based on an adult assessment. Marianne might have cried because she didn't understand why she would be given one object 'directly' while another was withheld. Perhaps she gradually learned to read her mother's facial expression and to trust her judgements.

Mothers usually want their babies to be outgoing and affectionate towards visitors. But Elizabeth, always a sensitive observer, considered the visitors from Marianne's perspective.

> *I do not think she is remarkably shy, although more so than she was. But certainly most people take children in such a brusque injudicious manner that no wonder they are often shy.*[39]

She couldn't change the way people treated Marianne, but the 'brusque injudicious manner' clearly jarred as it wasn't the sensitive way that she related to her child. However, she had noticed that it was how adults commonly related to children, and that this would make sense of children reacting by being 'shy'.

The first entry in her diary has an interesting ending:

> *I had no idea the journal of my disposition, & feelings was so intimately connected with that of my little baby, whose regular breathing has been the music of my thoughts all the time I have been writing. God bless her.*[40]

It is easy for a mother to focus on her child and almost forget her own existence. It sounds as though Elizabeth suddenly remembered herself as she prepared to stop writing. From this first entry in her diary, we can see that mother and daughter certainly were already 'intimately connected.' Marianne had laughed when her mother did, and her mother had cried when her daughter did. Six months in, the two of them were sharing their lives.

As a woman with several responsibilities besides motherhood, Elizabeth relied on the support of her servants. This gave her an emotional problem which she confronted with her usual honesty. Many mothers today will recognise it. She started by confessing: 'William told me the other day I was not of a jealous disposition; I do not think he knows me.' She then described Betsy, their faithful servant, who looked after her daughter some of the time. On one occasion Elizabeth recorded that Marianne, aged just over one year, seemed to prefer Betsy to her mother. Elizabeth found this hard, though she respected all that Betsy did. That was when she experienced the unchristian sense of jealousy. She managed to keep this so well hidden that her husband hadn't noticed. Instead, she comforted herself:

> *There will come a time when she* [Marianne] *will know how a mother's love exceeds all others; and meanwhile I will try never to put myself in rivalry with another for my child's affections.*[41]

Elizabeth was making a good point. She gave her love for her daughter as an ongoing and life-long commitment. The warmest and most hardworking servant is in a different position. She may love the child in her care but she is an employee who can be dismissed or, as happened to Betsy, recalled. Two years later, Betsy had to leave them as she was wanted by her own family after the death of a sister. But a mother cannot leave her young child in the same way. So Elizabeth was right to understand that she didn't need to rival her servant for her child's love. However, that didn't stop her from experiencing the pangs of jealousy. Mothers today who employ professional help to care for their children may well recognise that jealousy together with a similar sense of guilt.

Elizabeth loved truth and wanted Marianne to be confident that the adults around her would be truthful in what they told her. Several times in *My Diary*, she wrote that she made sure neither she nor her servants placated her daughter with impossible promises:

> *I have never allowed her to be told anyone was going to do anything for her, unless they really were, and have tried to speak as truly to her as ever I could.*[42]

The Old English word 'truth' is related to 'troth' and 'trust'. By being truthful, Elizabeth wanted Marianne to know that she could trust her mother and the people around her.

> *A trustful spirit on her* [Marianne's] *part can not be made by violence, but will come naturally when she sees that we* [Marianne's parents] *are scrupulous in respecting her little rights.*[43]

It's not clear what Marianne's 'little rights' were, but they must have included adults being honest with her, and not fobbing her off with false promises. However, truth didn't always mean 'the whole truth'. Later in *My Diary* Elizabeth explained that she edited the truth to fit what she thought her daughter could manage (see page 47).

As if this wasn't enough to think about, there was also Marianne's physical development. Elizabeth had a clear straightforward plan on this.

> *I intend that she* [Marianne] *shall teach herself to walk, & and receive no assistance from hands &c.*[44]

This was because

> *the more I see and hear of children the more I am convinced that when they feel their limbs strong enough to begin to walk they will constantly be trying their powers, & that till Nature prompts this, it is worse than useless to force them to their feet.*[45]

She was proved right. When Marianne was 22 months, 'she began, unexpectedly, to walk by herself.' It must have been an exciting moment for both of them.

In some ways, Elizabeth's values were typical of her society. She berated herself for not being patient enough. She was also sufficiently of her time to believe that a little girl should be taught to be patient, obedient, and in control of her passions. In her early years, Marianne failed to live up to these qualities. She sounds a lively, high-spirited little girl who didn't always do what she was told. When she was 'naughty' her parents resorted to ordering her to stand in a corner. But Marianne doesn't sound very penitent. She replied: '"I do [go] into a corner and be [a] naughty little girl."'[46] Typical of many children, Marianne was aware of being punished, but not of the intended message that the punishment was meant to teach her.

But her high spirits were exactly the kind of quality that contemporary parents were urged to suppress (in children, not in adults). One evening, her parents were teaching her to say her vowels. Marianne was then three years old. She knew her vowels but refused to say 'A'. So her parents felt that she had to be taught obedience.

> *Wm* [William] *gave her a slap on her hand every time she refused to say it, till at last she said it quite pat. Still, I am sure we were so unhappy that we cried, when she was gone to bed.*[47]

That is an interesting admission. Their tears indicate that both seemed to *feel* that there was something wrong in using force to compel their daughter to obey her father. But neither felt ready to disagree with it.

In other ways, Marianne sounds very much the daughter of both parents. Elizabeth records her saying when she was three: '"I love you, and Papa, & Meta [her baby sister], & Elizabeth & Fanny [two servants], and poor people.'[48] William Gaskell was a devoted Unitarian minister to some of the very poorest families in Manchester. And Elizabeth herself taught Sunday school classes at the Mosley Street Chapel. Ten years later, she published anonymously her first novel *Mary Barton* in which she gives a harrowing account of poverty in Manchester. Marianne had obviously sensed her parents' concern for those much poorer than themselves.

Elizabeth's beloved Aunt Lumb died on 1 May 1837 while

two-year-old Marianne was visiting her. However, even after almost a year had passed, Elizabeth still felt that Marianne was not yet ready to learn about death. This might have been because, some months earlier, when Marianne was just over two years old, she had seen a funeral while walking with Betsy. Betsy explained that it was 'a poor girl that they were going to put into a hole and cover her up with earth.'[49] Marianne must have been horrified. She woke up at night, talking about it. Elizabeth was able to calm her. But this is a perennial problem for parents when their child learns something frightening from another adult, not themselves. For Elizabeth, death was an ever-present possibility and an emotional subject. Surely she meant to tell Marianne about it herself, and from within a Christian context.

Mothers today are often troubled by how much to tell their children about illness and death. Elizabeth was truthful, but tactful too. Even though Marianne had witnessed the death of Aunt Lumb, Elizabeth wrote: 'We have never told her that Aunt Lumb was dead, fearing that a child's material ideas might connect gloom with the idea of one so blessed.'[50] Until Marianne was ready for the reality, Elizabeth assured her that: 'she [Aunt Lumb] is well and happy now' – an assurance that was consistent with the Gaskells' Unitarian faith. It's an example of how each mother has to judge for herself how much to explain to her young child.

She and Marianne discussed religion soon after she wrote that it was too soon for Marianne to learn about death. Elizabeth told her daughter that God loved her and watched over her at night. Marianne asked with a child's perplexity: '"When does – [i.e. God] go to bed."' It was a perfectly logical question, but Elizabeth was surprised by her daughter's 'material' ideas. She wrote: 'She [Marianne] has never asked any question whatever that could lead to any, even the most simple truths, of religion. I am on the watch for anything of that sort.'[51] On the watch she might be, as the wife of a minister, but careful not to suggest those kinds of questions if Marianne did not.

Elizabeth's third daughter, and the second to survive, Meta, was born on 5 February 1837, when Marianne was two years and five months old. It would have been a novel experience for Elizabeth. She probably had older sisters of her own, but they had died before she was born. She called some of her in-laws her 'sisters', but she had not grown up with them. She was familiar with siblings among her cousins. But watching sisterhood develop between her own two daughters must have shown her a very intimate relationship that she had never known.

Because they were both girls and close in age, it may have felt natural to compare them. This Elizabeth did, but in the spirit of wanting to understand how children could differ. She loved them both, so she tried to discover their individual qualities, but not with a view to setting them in competition with one another. What pleased her was that 'The two dear little sisters are very fond of one another.' She was amazed at how different they were in character. Even at 10 months, Elizabeth observed about Meta: 'I fancy she will be more clever than her elder sister, if not so gentle.'[52] It is typical of her that she balanced Meta's potential cleverness with Marianne's gentleness. It must have fascinated her to perceive that both girls were good – but in their own ways.

Her generosity towards differences in character will become significant in comparison with Fanny Nightingale, Florence's mother. Mrs Nightingale's two daughters were very different. Rather than enjoying both, she decided that Florence, unlike Parthenope, her older sister, was difficult to manage.

Elizabeth was to have four children who survived, all daughters. From the many letters she wrote to each of them as adults, it is clear that the warmth and trust she had built up with each daughter was mutual and lasting. 'My girls, my darlings *are* such comforts – such happiness,' she wrote in January 1860.[53] Marianne was by then 25, Meta nearly 23, Florence 17 and Julia 13. Elizabeth herself was 59, and had lost none of her love for the four of them.

The last entry of *My Diary* was for 28 October 1838. It doesn't have a formal ending. There might have been several reasons for not continuing. For example, at four, Marianne was now able to read. Elizabeth wanted to give her the diary, but perhaps not while she was in the middle of writing it. *My Diary* was probably meant to go on for longer. Yet she may have already said most of what she wanted.

Besides, looking after two little girls must have taken up a lot of her energy. She was also running her household and garden where she kept animals and grew vegetables at various times. She taught in Manchester, and she visited and wrote letters to her friends, and eventually published short stories and novels. Her first novel was published 10 years later, in 1848. *Mary Barton* was published under a pseudonym. It received immediate public attention. Readers were outspoken, both for and against its social content.

Looking at *My Diary* as a whole, what can we learn from it about motherhood? There are many more perceptive details in its pages than the short extracts used as examples here. So why has this work gone 'below the radar' of popular attention?

Elizabeth asked herself good questions, but she didn't have all the answers. If she thought that she had, *that* would have created interest *above* the radar. People seem to crave rules and certainties. She was surrounded by confident and didactic parenting books: not as many publications as there are today, but, in a similar way, each advocating a particular method and adding warnings of the evils that would befall the child if the mother did not follow it. Elizabeth's courage was in being able to admit, in a similar way to Socrates, how much others claimed to know, though she knew that she didn't know.

My Diary shows us that *how* to be a mother is not innate. It has to be learned. Many women can remember what their own mothers did so they have a model that they can copy. Elizabeth had to start from the beginning. For a responsible mother like herself, it was both daunting and exciting. She had to make daily decisions that she realised would affect her daughter when she was older.

Decisions like hers operate below the radar because they are silent ideas that mothers rarely discuss. But do they matter? Don't children outgrow their mothers' decisions? Many memoirs and autobiographies show how adults imbibed their mother's values when they were young, and continue to be affected by them. We encapsulate that process in the expression we use about learning 'at our mother's knee.' Elizabeth could see that some of her choices were taking effect, as for example making sure that neither she nor her servants promised her child anything that they couldn't fulfil. As a result, Marianne was evidently able to trust the word of the adults around her.

As we have seen, Elizabeth was silent about her experiences of pregnancy and childbirth. She mentions in one letter that she 'nursed' (i.e. breastfed) her son William, so probably she breastfed all her children. But we don't know for how long, nor whether she awoke at night to breastfeed while her babies were young. In 1854, she wrote to Parthenope that a mother local to Lea Hurst was unable to breastfeed on one side, and was feeding her baby on sago, 'which I disapproved of.'[54] Her reticence about the more physical side of mothering is curious, because, in her novels, she didn't flinch from many other 'unmentionable' subjects.

There is much more to *My Diary* than is relevant here. But perhaps these short extracts provide a sense of Elizabeth's understanding of motherhood, writing intimately only for herself (and eventually for Marianne). She wasn't writing for us. And it's interesting to note that, although Elizabeth was frequently terrified that Marianne might die, especially when she heard that other children nearby had died suddenly, she intended *My Diary* to be given to Marianne when she was older. So, along with her fears, Elizabeth seems to have had a degree of confidence that perhaps, after all, Marianne would survive.

In case Elizabeth sounds like a mother totally engrossed in her children and her home, she was clear that she was not. She clarified this in a letter she wrote to her friend Eliza Fox, dated around February 1850, and therefore just before the Gaskells moved house to Plymouth Grove:

> *I am sure it is healthy for them* [i.e. women] *to have the refuge of the hidden world of Art to shelter themselves in when too much pressed upon by daily small Lilliputian arrows of peddling cares; it... takes them into the land where King Arthur lies hidden, and soothes them with its peace. I have found this in writing.*[55]

By October 1854, when she came to Lea Hurst, her four daughters were much older. Marianne and Meta were then 20 and 17 years old, Florence was 12 and Julia eight. Elizabeth had begun writing professionally, submitting short stories and serialised novels to journals. To an aspiring writer, she wrote, years later:

> *When I had little children I do not think I could have written stories, because I should have become too much absorbed in my fictitious people to attend to my real ones.*[56]

However, Julia, her youngest child, was born on 3 September 1846. She would have been quite 'little' when Elizabeth started work on *Mary Barton*, published in October 1848. But by then she was an experienced mother. She may have been able to attend to Julia as well as write.

Elizabeth was able to use her mothering experiences in each of her novels. That includes the one she was writing at Lea Hurst. The early chapters of *North and South* had already been published as a serial in Dickens' journal, *Household Words* (see pp. 16–17). She knew how she wanted the novel to end. She wrote quickly, and needed to work on the middle chapters. So did she reach her ending at Lea Hurst? That was the plan, but there was so much happening in the house to distract her.

Chapter 4

Gaskell: 'If I could get over this next piece'

As Elizabeth became nationally well-known as a novelist, she was often invited to the homes of interested gentry. She enjoyed these visits. The Nightingales would have seemed just another of those gentry families that were glad to have her. Up till then, the family wasn't especially famous. That was a change that occurred very suddenly, during Elizabeth's visit. However, Elizabeth was a perceptive guest, and she didn't require national interest to realise what an exceptional person Florence was.

The letters she wrote from Lea Hurst show what an exciting visit she was having. It's incredible that she found enough time to work on the whole middle section of *North and South*, which was turning into a long novel, while also satisfying her enormous curiosity about Florence and the Nightingale family, and even finding time to describe them in detailed letters to her close friends.

Elizabeth must have needed courage to persevere with *North and South*. Her third novel, *Ruth*, had been published a year earlier. 'Of course you have read "Ruth" by this time,' wrote George Eliot to a friend on 1 February 1853, only a week or two after it had been published. This suggests how popular Elizabeth's work must have become.

Ruth was a 15-year-old who was seduced by an apparently charming gentleman. However, he abandoned her after getting her pregnant. Elizabeth made clear how much social stigma Ruth suffered, especially as she (Ruth) never named her seducer, so his reputation remained unsullied. Many readers wrote to praise the work. Florence Nightingale had enjoyed reading it.[1] But others were outraged by its supposedly scandalous subject matter, and

Elizabeth became ill, soon after its publication, with what she called 'a "Ruth" fever'.

> *Oh! I was so poorly! And cd not get over the hard things that people said of* Ruth. *I mean I was just in that feverish way when I could not get them out of my head… I do so manage to shock people… Yet two men have* [burnt their copies of *Ruth*]; *and a third has forbidden his wife to read it; they sit next to us in* [Cross Street] *Chapel and you can't think how 'improper' I feel under their eyes.*[2]

It must have been reassuring when Charles Dickens offered to publish her next work as a serial in his weekly journal, *Household Words*. He had launched the journal in 1850. It was to contain literature of general interest, and to retail at the affordable price of 2d (two old pence) a copy. He had got to know Elizabeth about six years earlier when she sent him a copy of her first novel, *Mary Barton*. He was quick to recognise her outstanding ability as a writer. So, in 1850, when he was planning *Household Words,* Elizabeth seems to have been the first writer he approached to contribute to his new project. In January 1850, he wrote to her:

> *there is no living English writer whose aid I would desire to enlist in preference to the author of* Mary Barton *(a book that profoundly affected and impressed me). I venture to ask you whether you can give me any hope that you will write a short tale, or any number of tales, for the projected pages.*[3]

He must have been determined to engage her, because he offered to visit her in Manchester to discuss his proposal further. She accepted his offer and wrote several stories for him. Her second novel, *Cranford*, was first published in *Household Words*, in several episodes.

As well as the 'grand quarrel' that Elizabeth was soon to have with Florence Nightingale, she was having a painful dispute with

Dickens about the length of *North and South*. They had both won national fame as novelists. Dickens was the more popular, and soon became aware of what seemed to be Elizabeth's insecurity about herself as a writer. He complained:

> *If you weren't the most suspicious of women, always looking for soft sawder* [flattery] *in the purest metal of praise, I should call your paper delightful and touching in the tenderest and most delicate manner. Being what you are, I confine myself to the observation that I have called it 'A Love Affair at Cranford' and sent it off to the printer.*[4]

However, Elizabeth wasn't at all 'suspicious' of all praise. Dickens lavished extravagant compliments on her work, that she, being keen on exact truth, might have found excessive. He knew her work was an asset to *Household Words* and needed to retain her. But he also held criticisms that he revealed to his sub-editor (page 55) but not to her. She was sensitive, so she may well have felt unsure of him.

In *North and South*, Gaskell was hoping to reconcile some of the social disparities she had described in *Mary Barton*. She needed to tread carefully. Her new novel had a romantic theme, but she also wanted her readers to think about their divided society, without being roused to the polarised positions they had taken in response to her earlier works. 'If only I have made people talk & discuss the subject a little more than they did,' was her aim.[5] But by now she knew how quickly her readers' emotions could be inflamed. 'No one can feel more deeply than I how wicked it is to do anything to excite class against class,' she wrote.[6]

She sent the first part of *North and South* to Dickens in June 1854. Fortunately, he wrote back in approval:

> *It opens an admirable story, is full of character and power, has a strong suspended interest in it (the end of which I don't in the least foresee), and has the very best marks of your hand upon it.*[7]

Dickens advertised the serial in advance. In July, he announced that the first chapters would come out in *Household Words* in September. At the end of each instalment, he advertised the next ones for the following week. He published two, and occasionally three, chapters at a time. But he hadn't got the whole novel. In July, he wrote: 'The fifth part to end with the end of the Thornton declaration scene, and the end of the MS I have.'[8] The 'Thornton declaration scene' occurs in Chapter 24, which Dickens published with chapters 25 and 26 on 25 November 1854. So, in October, while Elizabeth was staying at Lea Hurst, Dickens must have been impatient for the rest.

However, their interests diverged. Dickens wanted a fast-moving serial by this famous author to attract more readers to *Household Words*. But Elizabeth was writing a story that grew, once she had started, and unfolded slowly as she started to develop the details of her main characters. She had the difficult task of conveying, through them, a serious social message in serial form, and keeping readers interested from week to week.

By 20 August, Dickens had already complained that some of her early dialogues were too long, and asked her to make cuts. On 14 October, unbeknown to her and while she was at Lea Hurst, Dickens wrote to his sub-editor that he was sorry to hear of the drop in the sales of *Household Words*, but was not surprised as 'Mrs Gaskell's story, so divided, is wearisome in the last degree.'[9]

A power struggle had arisen between them and it's interesting that each thought the other had won. Dickens resented the length of the final chapters, but he couldn't truncate the novel prematurely. Grudgingly, he had to allow Elizabeth two extra issues of *Household Words* to bring the story to its conclusion. Elizabeth felt she had been forced to hurry and that pressure from Dickens had ruined what was to have been a much better novel. 'Indeed I do not like writing a *long* story,' she wrote to Harriet Martineau, another brilliant writer, 'to be broken up into little bits in a serial publication.'[10]

At a casual glance, this seems to have been a second grand

quarrel – this time between Elizabeth and Dickens. They were certainly angry with one another. She was determined never to write for him again. But theirs was a professional relationship and they were able to mend it. For Elizabeth, this ongoing but more negotiable quarrel must have simmered in the background of her dispute with Florence Nightingale.

She didn't finish *North and South* at Lea Hurst. But she seems to have written fast. At first she sounds delighted with what she had achieved. 'I do think she [Margaret Hale, the main character in *North and South*] is going on well. I am satisfied. Not that I have written so much but so *well*.'[11]

It's worth looking at *North and South*, both to reveal what Elizabeth used from her experience as a mother, and also how she was influenced by her stay at Lea Hurst.

The novel starts in the south of England, where Margaret Hale lives with her parents, before they all move to the north. Here Margaret makes friends with a mill-worker and his sick daughter. But her position is an independent one. She is interested in the mill owners as well as their workers. Through the character of Margaret, Elizabeth was able to analyse the critical social divisions from both sides.

Margaret and her parents are invited to a party given by Mrs Thornton, the mother of John Thornton, one of the rich mill owners. Margaret discusses the party invitation with Bessie, the sick daughter of a mill-worker. Bessie is awed at the prospect of the party. She says to Margaret in her Lancashire dialect: 'yo' see, they thinken a deal o' money here, and I reckon yo've not gotten much.' Margaret agrees that her family is poor. 'But we are educated people and have lived among educated people,' she replies.[12] This seems to have been Elizabeth's position too.

Margaret is able to enjoy the company of mill owners and mill workers alike. She goes to the Thornton party with her father, and finds herself listening to the men's conversation. Elizabeth distinguishes her from the other women there who have more trivial concerns:

> *There was a very animated conversation going on among the gentlemen; the ladies, for the most part, were silent, employing themselves in taking notes of the dinner and criticising each other's dresses. Margaret caught the clue to the general conversation, grew interested, and listened attentively.*[13]

Margaret's ability to listen reminds us again of Elizabeth. And Florence, who read these chapters months later in *Household Words* at Scutari, would surely have understood Margaret's interest in serious male conversation. Her own early social experiences were very like those of the fictional Margaret's.

The character of Margaret Hale develops during the novel. She sounds similar to Elizabeth in the chapters written before Lea Hurst. After that, Margaret slowly becomes more like Florence Nightingale. She grows more independent, more religious, more determined not to marry, and more conscious of her moral failings. Elizabeth also describes her beauty in language very similar to the terms she uses in a letter praising the beauty of Florence.

Elizabeth contrasted two mothers in *North and South*. Both love their children, but in different ways. Mrs Hale, Margaret's mother, is presented as decent but weak. Her daughter has to care for her, rather than the usual way round. What a contrast to Mrs Thornton, mother of the mill owner John Thornton. Mrs Thornton seems cold but strong, and very supportive of her son. Elizabeth uses small details to develop both characters. Neither mother is idealised. Mrs Hale has relatively little influence on the unfolding story, but Mrs Thornton's strong feelings for her son affect the entire plot. These sections were almost certainly written at Lea Hurst, and show how profoundly Elizabeth was concerned with the influence of mothers at about the time of her dispute with Florence Nightingale.

Mrs Hale is unable to cope with the move from the south of England to the north. She eventually sickens and dies. Near the end of her character's life, Elizabeth slips in a very unattractive detail. She has Mrs Hale confess to her daughter that she had once preferred her son, Frederick. She tells Margaret that he was a beautiful baby whereas Margaret was 'an ugly little thing.'[14] Margaret doesn't seem to object to this early description of herself. But readers of *My Diary* would know how fairly Elizabeth treated her own four children. She saw individual goodness in each, and it's difficult to imagine her preferring one, or considering any of them 'ugly'. She doesn't comment on Mrs Hale's admission, but allows readers to judge for themselves.

As we know, Dickens had received all the chapters up to the 'Thornton declaration' scene. In this scene, Thornton makes a passionate declaration of love to Margaret. She refuses him, and he is devastated. Unable to bear returning straight home, he gets on a bus that carries him out of the city.

Elizabeth leaves Thornton in torment, and unexpectedly takes her readers into the dining-room of his house where his mother sits, waiting for him. Readers know that he has been rejected by Margaret, but his mother does not. It never occurs to her that her beloved son could be anything but accepted. She imagines that he is late coming home because he is having such a delightful time with his bride-to-be. Soon there will be another Mrs Thornton, she supposes, and she will be supplanted. What will this mean? Her ideas are practical. She decides: 'The newly-wed couple would need fresh household stocks of linen.' She has baskets of tablecloths and napkins brought to her. Some are marked GHT for George (her deceased husband) and Hannah (herself) Thornton.

> *Some... were Dutch damask of the old kind, exquisitely fine; none were like them now. Mrs Thornton stood looking at them long; they had been her pride when she was first married. Then she knit her brows, and pinched and compressed her lips tight, and carefully unpicked the GH. She went so far as to search for the Turkey red marking-thread to put in the new initials, but it was all used – and she had no heart to send for any more, just yet.*[15]

We immediately get the sense of a decisive woman, able to follow through with compressed lips a painful choice, however much it hurt her. And it's curious that there was no need to include this scene. The plot didn't require it. Anyone who had read this far would already know Margaret's character. It would be obvious that, even if Margaret had accepted Thornton, she wouldn't be interested in initialled table linen. The scene isn't even significant in showing how Mrs Thornton affected the unfolding main plot. That whole sequence comes later. So this scene allows readers to see a different side to Mrs Thornton, a curious insight into her character. Usually Mrs Thornton is presented as cold and unsympathetic. But here Elizabeth reveals her vulnerability in an intimate detail, and it's difficult not to feel a degree of pity for her.

So far, Elizabeth had made good progress with *North and South*. However, a few days after writing that the story was 'going on well' and that she was satisfied with it, she wrote another letter to her friend, Emily Shaen, and confessed that she wasn't sure how to continue. She had planned the ending, but wasn't sure how to reach it. Her letter was written just hours before she left Lea Hurst, and sounds, for a woman who wrote as clearly as she did, oddly incoherent.

> *I've got to (with Margaret Hale – I'm off at her now following your letter) when they've quarrelled, silently, after he* [Mr Thornton] *and she knows she loves him, and he is trying not to love her; and Frederick* [Margaret's brother] *is gone back to Spain and Mrs Hale is dead and Mr Bell* [Margaret's godfather] *has come to stay with the Hales, and Mr Thornton ought to be developing himself – and Mr Hale ought to die – and if I could get over this next piece I could swim through the London life beautifully into the sunset glory of the last scene.*[16]

Mr Bell, Margaret's godfather, visits the Hales in Chapter 40, so Gaskell must have been writing at great speed. But here she sounds stuck. If *North and South* wasn't being serialised, she could have put it aside until more ideas came to her. Eventually, she managed to send Dickens another 16 long chapters. 'Every page was grudged me,' she complained to her friend and author Anna Jameson.[17] On 17 December, she sent Dickens 33 further pages. She wrote to him:

> *I can only feel depressed by it* [North and South], *so what I send today is meant to be crammed and stuffed into Janry 20th* [of *Household Words*]; *& I'm afraid I've nearly as much more the Janry 27th* [the final date Dickens had allowed her for her serial. She knew he thought the novel too long, and gave him permission to shorten it.] *Don't consult me as to the shortenings, only please yourself.'*[18]

That sounds like an admission of defeat. She wrote to Anna Jameson again: 'If the story had been poured just warm out of the mind, it would have taken a much larger mould. It was the cruel necessity of compressing it that hampered me.'[19] Jameson was shocked and replied:

> *It enrages me to lose that beautiful picture of the gradual opening of the mutual mind and heart of the two beings you have created with such intense vitality and which you would have given such delicacy and power – so here you have my opinion most crudely and unceremoniously but most truly.*[20]

Jameson seems to be saying: How could you let Dickens shorten your work? Why didn't you stand up to him?

Elizabeth had a book contract and, once the serialisation was printed, the novel came out complete in two volumes. She wrote an introductory note explaining that she had added some extra chapters near the end. But readers may still find the actual ending sudden and abrupt.

Something of the confidence and delight she had experienced when first writing at Lea Hurst had deserted her. Yet Charlotte Brontë admired the serialised *North and South.*[21] And a second edition of the two-volume book was published soon after the first. It was translated into French and German, and published in America. There doesn't seem to be an original manuscript, so we can't tell what Dickens had cut. Yet, between them, they had produced a successful novel.

Elizabeth blamed Dickens for not allowing her the freedom to make her novel as long as she wanted. But Dickens had been urging her to shorten her work long before she reached the last chapters. She could have protested. He was committed to publishing her in *Household Words*, and could surely have shifted more contributions to make extra room for her, if she had insisted.

Something seems to have occurred at Lea Hurst to lessen her confidence. In the next chapter, we shall see how profoundly she admired Florence Nightingale. It was during Elizabeth's visit that Florence learned that the War Office would fund her to take a team of nurses to Scutari. Now there would be nurses to interview and much to prepare. Elizabeth heard Florence say that: 'She never reads any book now. She has not time for it, to begin with; and secondly she says life is so vivid that books seem poor.'[22] It seems a tactless remark for Florence to have made in the hearing of her mother's guest who had come to write her novel in their house. Elizabeth does not say how she felt on hearing this. But she quoted it and must have been affected, as she was sensitive and easily hurt.

When Elizabeth arrived at Lea Hurst, Florence was staying there on an extended holiday from her hospital work, so Elizabeth had a good opportunity to get to know her. She was filled with admiration. 'She is like a saint,' was one of her first impressions, written to her friend Catherine Winkworth. 'Is it not like St Elizabeth of Hungary?'[23] It's interesting that they both knew of St Elizabeth, an early medieval saint best known for her charitable works.

Their grand quarrel seems to have occurred at about this time. Elizabeth doesn't give an exact date. We will come to it in Chapter 7 after considering Florence and the contrasting experiences that she brought to it. When the Nightingale family hurried to London, Elizabeth was desperately curious to learn what happened next.

She wrote to Parthenope a few days later, asking for news of the family. She apologised for wanting information at such a busy time, adding that she asked 'as a beggar' who had no claim to information. Although she read the newspapers, they didn't tell her 'what I am so greedy to know.'[24]

During the first part of her stay at Lea Hurst, Elizabeth enjoyed the care of an excellent hostess. Fanny Nightingale, born in 1788, was just old enough to have been Elizabeth's mother. It's easy to see her as superficial through the angry words of her rebellious younger daughter. But Elizabeth experienced a different side of her. Mrs Nightingale found time to talk to her interesting guest, who must have been an eager listener. Through Mrs Nightingale, Elizabeth learned exactly those early details that she wanted to know about Florence.

Yet even Elizabeth, sensitive to mothers as she was, gives *no* description of Mrs Nightingale herself. She wrote lively and very perceptive portraits of Parthenope and Florence. She described a little of Mr Nightingale and introduced him as 'a *very* superior man.'[25] But of Mrs Nightingale we only hear: 'Mrs N. tells me...' and 'Mrs N. says...'.[26]

> *She* [Florence] *had the toothache, and an abscess in her mouth, and Mrs N. was very anxious about her, as she was evidently not strong. On Monday she said, 'I am going* [to London] *tomorrow.' This took them quite by surprise as she evidently was still very poorly; and Mrs N. remonstrated. But it turned out she had written and made so many arrangements depending on her presence, before she had even spoken about it to her family, that they had nothing to do but to yield.*[27]

Frances Nightingale, an adventurous woman once famous for her vivacity and beauty, seems to have no individual identity in Elizabeth's letters, apart from being an excellent hostess and anecdote-telling mother. This must have been deliberate, though there is no clue as to the reason. However, Elizabeth appreciated the care taken of her.[28] And she seems to have retained warm feelings for Mrs Nightingale because she wrote a quick note four months later saying: 'Mrs Nightingale Only passing thro' London very sorry not to see you.'[29] She wasn't in the habit of writing quick apologetic notes, so this presumably means that she wasn't indifferent to her hostess. But she says nothing whatsoever about the impression Mrs Nightingale made on her. As a mother and author, she must have formed some idea of Mrs Nightingale's character. But we are left with quite a pointed and tantalising silence.

However, once the family had left, Elizabeth seems to have felt lonely and restless. She liked to hear the voices of people talking, rather than being marooned in her room in order to write. She had refused formal invitations to visit local gentry friends, but she walked to several neighbouring cottages and chatted to the women who lived there. She wrote to Parthenope: 'Then to Mrs Storer's where I sate some time, making her husband's acquaintance, & hearing a deal about the lead mines.'[30] She loved listening to technical details, and this is a typical example of one of the ways she collected descriptions that she could use in a novel. But perhaps she was also seeking out company because she felt abandoned once the family had gone.

She must surely have felt unsettled by her quarrel with Florence. Now she had no opportunity to discuss the issues further and to restore their friendly relationship. And she, who missed her own mother so much, would also have felt the maternal care of Mrs Nightingale. It may have given her a precious sense of security. She was freed from her usual practical responsibilities. At last she could concentrate on keeping track of all the strands that made up the complicated plot of *North and South*. But very likely the large silent house didn't feel the same without its family. She had two secluded rooms with coal and candles. Yet Elizabeth needed people, and managed to write in her living room at home, with family and friends present and talking. Sustained by the company of the Nightingale family, perhaps she would have found the strength to tackle Dickens.

She was invited to stay for as long as she wanted to finish the novel. But she only stayed a week longer than the family. On 27 October she left, with *North and South* still far from her planned ending.

Chapter 5

Nightingale: 'I have no desire now but to die'

Florence Nightingale was 30 years old when she confessed in a private note that she wanted to die. She was a vivacious, well-educated, well-connected young woman from a wealthy family. How could she have become so unhappy?

In 1851, she wrote to her mother: 'I sh'd be as happy here as the day is long & wish I could hope that I had your smile, your blessing, your sympathy upon it – without which I cannot be quite happy.'[1] It doesn't sound much to ask from a mother. What had gone wrong? 'Oh, dear good woman,' she wrote about her mother in a private note to herself, 'when I feel her disappointment in me, it is as if I was becoming insane.'[2]

Why did Florence feel her mother was disappointed in her? They were two strong-willed women who could not agree. Mrs Nightingale's outlook was adventurous but more conventional. Florence could see her mother's viewpoint only too well. 'When she has organised the nicest Society in England for us, & I cannot take it as she wishes.'[3] 'Us' meant herself and her sister. Her sister evidently could take 'it', meaning that Parthenope enjoyed the many parties of cultured upper-class guests that her mother would arrange. 'She [Parthenope] is in union with her age,' observed Florence.[4] By 'her age', Florence must have meant their generation of young women who appreciated these parties. By all appearances, Florence enjoyed them too, and Parthenope felt jealous that she could not match the vivacity of her younger sister. In private, however, Florence protested that elegant parties weren't what she wanted, but neither Mrs Nightingale nor Parthenope seems to have understood or sympathised with her.

Fanny or Frances Smith – the future Mrs Nightingale – had grown up as the fourth of 10 siblings in a lively family. She was the third girl, so perhaps she received mothering from her older sisters and an aunt, as well as from her mother. It could well have looked to her as though the 10 of them looked after one other and didn't need much motherly care. Mrs Nightingale's parents, Frances and William Smith, enjoyed travelling for pleasure for months at a time, using an open phaeton, exploring castles and beautiful views in England, Wales and Scotland. Having children didn't curtail their style. They took their growing family with them. All 10 siblings seem to have thrived on adventure and travel, and survived to adulthood, which was unusual at a time when many died young. In the year that Fanny was born, 1788, her parents crossed the Channel to France. They visited Paris and Versailles, as both parents (Florence's maternal grandparents) loved art. Her grandfather, William Smith, collected artworks and became a founder member of the National Gallery in London. Fanny must have grown up to take long journeys for granted, and was surely accustomed to the clip-clop rhythm of horse's hooves and the rumble of phaeton wheels, either when she was in the womb or as a young child. This influence becomes important when she grew up and married.

She married William Nightingale, six years younger than herself, in 1818. The Napoleonic Wars had ended with the Battle of Waterloo three years earlier, which meant that Europe was safe again for English travellers. The Nightingales took advantage of this. They both enjoyed travelling, and the excitement of seeing famous views and art galleries. They got as far as Italy, which Fanny's mother had always longed to visit. They travelled south, reached Naples and rented a house, where their first child was born on 19 April 1819. Giving birth in Naples might sound straightforward today when the city is a short air-flight from England. But it had taken weeks of horse-and-carriage riding to get there. Even for a woman who had grown up travelling with her childhood family, it was risky. It was a romantic place, but not healthy, rife with known diseases, such as cholera, typhus and malaria. As for giving birth, Fanny's mother usually had an unmarried sister on call when her children were born. This was Fanny's first birth, and she wasn't young. She would have been about 30, with her sisters far off in England, and unable to give her practical support. After the birth a sister would have been especially valuable as the newborn was small and frail. Fanny knew two of her sisters had breastfed. She tried to breastfeed but found she couldn't produce enough milk.

Breastfeeding succeeds with a bit of experimenting and in a calm atmosphere, without panic. The usual problem, then as now, is about positioning. As the newborn was small, and Fanny quite tall, Fanny would have needed to hold her baby high enough for the baby to suck not just her nipple but a portion of her areola, to stimulate her milk supply. Fanny might not have known this, and the whole experience was frightening and humiliating for her. She could see that her daughter was failing to thrive, and understandably she panicked. In addition, she and her husband both became unwell. She wanted to breastfeed, but in the end resorted to a wet nurse.

At least she could choose a good name for her daughter. At a time when children were called after their parents, and there were confusing numbers of Annes, Marys, Elizabeths and Hannahs, Fanny first named her daughter Frances after herself and her own mother. Then she discovered an old name for Naples, Parthenope. She liked it, and gave it to her daughter as a middle name, but it soon became the name by which she was always known. Perhaps Fanny intended friends to ask: 'Why is she called Parthenope? My dear, you gave birth in *Naples*? I can scarcely believe it. How very brave of you. So far from home.' It had surely been a risky adventure. However, as the daughter of adventurous parents, she could feel vindicated in that she, her husband and Parthenope had all survived it.

Fanny became pregnant again only a few months later, which sounds very soon, given that she had been ill after Parthenope's birth. This time, the family travelled north, and rented a house on the outskirts of Florence. A second daughter was born on 12 May 1820. She, too, was named after the city of her birth, this time using the English name, Florence. Understandably, Fanny didn't want to go through the distress of attempting to breastfeed again, so Florence, like Parthenope, was fed by an Italian wet nurse.

This early history is important, as it may explain some of the difficulties that Florence experienced with her mother. In a notebook that she started when she was eight years old, written in French, which seems to have come easily to her, she started an autobiography. She translated her surname as 'Rossignol' (Nightingale). She recorded that she had been born in Florence, and had been given to a *balia* (wet nurse) as her mother had been too ill to nurse her. This notebook seems to have disappeared, but fortunately it was seen and cited by I.B. O'Malley in *Florence Nightingale 1820-1856*.[5] It seems that being nursed by a *balia* rather than her mother was important to eight-year-old Florence. She knew her mother had tried to breastfeed her sister. But, in her case, it seemed that her mother was too ill to try.

Florence's father had inherited the property of Lea Hall, then a modest farm house. It was entailed to a male heir, which meant that, when he died, Fanny, Parthenope and Florence would be rendered homeless, as they would be unable to inherit it. Obviously the situation would be resolved if Fanny could give birth to a son. But she didn't bear a third child.

The family returned to England in 1821. Mr Nightingale, with his inherited wealth, bought more land in Derbyshire. He designed and had built Lea Hurst, which was modest by gentry standards, but enabled the family to entertain. A drawback was that, after Italy, it felt very damp and cold, especially in winter. It was far from London, if they wanted to attract city guests, and there was not much hunting, shooting or fishing to be had. Fortunately, Mr Nightingale found a second, larger property in Embley Park in Hampshire, within easier reach from London, and with potential for hunting and shooting parties. It also adjoined the property of Lord Palmerston, who became a frequent visitor. He was the

British foreign minister for several years before serving as prime minister in 1855–58 and 1859–65. This must have helped Mrs Nightingale to make further aristocratic connections. Lea Hurst in Derbyshire was used for more intimate gatherings of writers, scientists, mathematicians, and politicians. Elizabeth's description of a typical Lea Hurst gathering is on page 18.

When Florence wrote about her mother: 'When she has organised the nicest Society in England for us…', it was no exaggeration. Within a few years, Fanny had 'networked' through the English aristocracy, including dukes and lords, and selected those she found interesting. She herself became a brilliant hostess, well-prepared and sociable. Her husband tended to be studious but more withdrawn. Guests enjoyed talking to him, but he needed drawing out and to be convinced that his guest was genuinely interested in his ideas. He helped to found the British Association for the Advancement of Science. He recognised the importance of statistics, and befriended the brilliant polymath Charles Babbage, who was pioneering the use of statistics. Mr Nightingale had travelled across Europe and met other leading scientists. Their discussions were serious. The ability to be as light and sociable as his wife was not his strong point.

Fanny could enter her drawing-room and bring her many diverse guests together in lively, enjoyable conversations. She was supported by a well-organised team of domestic staff that had been properly trained to her own high standard. She was one of 10 siblings, and must have seen her parents planning whole-family expeditions on a large scale. Fanny, too, could predict what her guests needed, both on a large scale, and in detail (as with coals and candles for Elizabeth Gaskell's visit), so that her hospitality ran smoothly and imperceptibly. When she was older, Florence said she felt frustrated at her mother's constant requests that she should go to the drawing room and entertain 'the nicest Society in England', but she must have absorbed how well her mother managed. Florence's ability to order supplies from England for the vast hospitals at Scutari, a prospect which would have daunted most people, was perhaps made easier for Florence, having grown up listening to her capable mother interviewing prospective staff members, organising them, and ordering whatever she thought each guest would need for a comfortable stay at her homes.

From a young age, Florence seems to have developed a sense of her own importance. She was unusual, and her family recounted stories about her. Florence herself remembered that, when she was six, she was sent downstairs to be diagnosed by the family doctor at Lea Hurst with whooping cough. 'Her thirteen dolls had it too,' recalled Parthenope, '& were found with pieces of flannel around 13 necks.'[6] Elizabeth was told 'of her 18 dolls all ill in rows in beds, when she was quite a little thing.'[7] So already, at only six years old, Florence had imagined herself nursing, not one-to-one, but on a large scale far beyond her young experience.

As a member of the local gentry, Mrs Fanny Nightingale would visit the sick in the villages round Lea Hurst, bringing soups, jellies and puddings, and offering comfort. Perhaps both daughters accompanied her on these visits, but people like the local journalist Llewellyn Hewitt remembered Florence especially. Florence would continue visiting even without her mother. Elizabeth discovered this when she walked round the cottages that neighboured Lea Hurst: 'She [Florence] used to go a great deal among the villagers here, who dote upon her.'[8]

It would be easy to assume that the Nightingales lived together, when they weren't entertaining, as a cosy foursome. Many families in their circles did exactly that. But both Nightingale parents were restless. Mr Nightingale liked to spend time in London, and also had to oversee his two estates at Lea Hurst and Embley. Fanny Nightingale was constantly travelling, to 'network', as we would say now, for her next house parties, or to visit friends, or to be useful to one of her siblings. She would send her daughters to stay with their cousins, or in exchange have their cousins stay with them, especially the Nicholsons and the Bonham Carters. Parthenope was delicate, and Fanny would order regimes for the health of both daughters, usually issued to their nurse or governess. However, she sounds as if she would have been impatient at spending too long a time with them herself. So Florence grew up in the lively society of her childhood cousins, much as Fanny had grown up with her siblings. This would have been significant when Florence started to form her own views on the role of mothers. There seems a distance between Florence and her mother, a lack of friendly intimacy. Florence received more motherly attention from her father's younger sister, her Aunt Mai. All this must have contributed to the idea she was to share with Elizabeth Gaskell.

Some of the details of Florence's childhood might yet be unknown, but for the letters Elizabeth wrote during her visit. She learned stories from Mrs Nightingale that fascinated her. While at Lea Hurst, she wrote to her friend Catherine Winkworth:

> *Mrs N. told me that when a girl of 15 or so she* [Florence] *was often missing in the evening, & Mrs N. would take a lantern & go up into the village to find her, sitting by the bedside of someone who was ill, & saying that she cd not sit down to a grand 7 o'clock dinner while &c.*[9]

And these dinners were completely unchanged by the time Elizabeth wrote. It's amazing to notice that, halfway through this same letter, Elizabeth interrupted her writing to tell her friend: 'Now I must go & dress for dinner. We dine at 7.'

But did Elizabeth appreciate what an act of rebellion it must have been for the teenage Florence to be missing in the evening when it was time to sit down to dinner? In her book *Cassandra*, Florence railed against the quasi-religious importance with which this ritual was observed:

> *Dinner is that great sacred ceremony of this day, the great sacrament. To be absent from dinner is equivalent to being ill. Nothing will excuse us from it. Bodily incapacity is the only apology valid.*[10]

When Florence was 30 and evidently bored and depressed, her parents arranged for their friends, the Bracebridges, to take her on a tour to Egypt and Athens. Elizabeth reported: 'Mrs N. says they [the Nightingales] equipped her *en princesse*, and when she came back she had little besides the clothes she wore; she had given away her linen & right & left to those who wanted it.'[11]

Mrs Nightingale presented a very positive picture of Florence to her guest. However, she didn't explain that, before then, she had found her younger daughter troublesome and intractable. It's not clear whether Elizabeth realised this. The two sisters, so close in age, were very different in character. A study of Florence's writing shows that she felt her ambitions were constantly thwarted by her mother. Her mother intended her to marry, and couldn't understand why Florence would want any other kind of life. By the time Mrs Nightingale was praising Florence to Elizabeth, she was also supporting her daughter in practical ways, and continued to do this during and after the Crimean War. But by then it was too late to redeem their relationship. Florence craved her mother's love and approval. It's clear that she never felt that she had it. Years later, when Florence was living alone (with a very efficient staff of servants) in South Street, London, she wrote a revealing note to her mother, dated 28 July 1865:

> *Dearest Mum – I hardly know what to say to your coming tomorrow. Even ten minutes' talk with those I love best secures me a night of agony and a week of feverish exhaustion... But if you would come up so as to be here about 4.00, and just come in and kiss me, that would be a great delight. But there must be no talk...*[12]

Florence had always been single-minded. She believed she had heard several calls from God assuring her that she was destined for divine work. The first call, she said, came to her on 7 February 1837, so she was then only 16. Yet even as a young child, she had a clear idea of what she wanted to do.

> *The first idea I can recollect when I was a child was a desire to nurse the sick. My daydreams were all of hospitals and I visited them whenever I could. I never communicated it to anyone – it would have been laughed at – but I thought God had called me to serve in that way.*[13]

Everyone in her family knew they could call on Florence when they were ill, and she would be capable of nursing them, often back to health. But this was respectable and quite different from aiming to become a professional nurse.

Her parents didn't laugh when she finally told them. They were horrified. They had heard that nurses were habitually drunk, dirty and incompetent. They were working-class women, more like cleaners than involved in patient care. Hospitals were known to be dangerous places where diseases spread, to the extent that even poor people avoided them.

Florence's first plan was to get some practical nursing experience by visiting Salisbury Infirmary during a period spent at the family's larger house nearby at Embley Park. When she revealed this plan to her parents, they were aghast. Her mother protested that Florence couldn't know what she would be letting herself in for. She might encounter a patient suffering from diseases that a lady could not think of, and certainly not mention. And she might be exposed to the attentions of surgeons who were not 'gentlemen'.

In despair, Florence wrote to her cousin, Hilary Bonham Carter: 'But there have been difficulties about my very first step [to learn nursing at Salisbury], which terrified Mama. I do not mean the physically revolting parts of a hospital but things about the surgeons and nurses which you may guess.'[14] It's not clear what Mr Nightingale thought. Though he had taught Florence so brilliantly, she complained about him in an unpublished note, especially of his 'utter indifference to me. He never cared *what I was* or what *I might become.*'[15] So Mrs Nightingale's opposition carried the day.

Without parental support, Florence did not see how she could progress. She was already 25, and thrown into desperation by her inability to carry out even this simple plan. She felt that she was being forced to make do with 'excitement', preparing for and attending the social events that were supposed to fulfil her, instead of pursuing a meaningful 'occupation': doing valuable work for others, for which she would need to be trained. She drew a significant comparison between the two:

> *I wish to show how twenty years of doing nothing, of living without occupation and by excitement, may cause to deteriorate the human brain to such an extent that I solemnly declare (after some experience in lunatics) I consider the people in Hanwell* [lunatic asylum in Middlesex] *who conceive themselves to be teapots, or to have 30,000 men fighting in their insides, to be not more the subject of delusions than the class which thus lives by excitement and not by occupation.*[16]

When there is no escape from a restrictive daily life, resorting to daydreams is a natural response. Florence was deeply ashamed of her daydreaming habit. She had been daydreaming for years, and felt it was sinful. Surely God would not trust His divine plan to a sinful woman like herself. Every so often, she recorded that she had 'cured' herself of daydreaming, but the habit returned and depressed her. She worried constantly that other people would notice. Certainly the observant Elizabeth seems to have witnessed it more than once during her visit to Lea Hurst. She wrote:

> *She* [Florence] *used to sit with her head bent a little forwards, one hand lying in repose over thc other on her knees looking in that steady way which means that people are not seeing the real actual before them.*[17]

Mrs Nightingale recognised that her younger daughter needed more to occupy her, and put her in charge of the still-room, the linen room, and the china cupboard at Lea Hurst. The still-room would be something like a large cool larder, containing stored foods. The linen room and china cupboard must have been to accommodate guests who were staying at Lea Hurst, where the servants would be ordered to launder their bedding and to bring out fine china to serve their meals. In retrospect, responsibility for these items of hospitality seems an excellent experience for a future hospital superintendent. Florence enjoyed organising these collections, though she puzzled: 'I cannot help thinking in my head. Can reasonable people want all this?'[18] But she also took the opportunity to be up before the rest of her family and, in the privacy of these rooms, she secretly studied hospital reports, sent to her by her friends.

Florence's more ambitious plan was to study at Kaiserswerth in Germany, where she had heard that nurses could be trained. With her friends, on returning from Cairo and Athens through Germany, she managed to pay a two-week visit to Kaiserswerth in the summer of 1850. There wasn't much practical training to be had, but her stay there delighted her, and gave her a sense of her own independence. She also realised how much potential there could be if nurses were properly trained. In a letter of 1852, she wrote:

> *It* [Kaiserswerth] *is first rate. I wish the system could be introduced in England, where thousands of women here have nothing to do and where hospitals are ill nursed by a class of women not fit to be household servants.*[19]

When Mrs Nightingale found out that Florence had visited Kaiserswerth she was furious. One dread she had was that if it became widely known that her younger daughter wanted to train to become a hospital nurse, this would amount to a family scandal that would ruin her older daughter's chances of a respectable marriage. No suitor had yet come forward to bid for Parthenope, though Florence had turned down at least two serious marriage proposals. Fanny Nightingale must have felt bound to put no impediment in the way of a gentleman proposing to Parthenope.

No wonder, then, that Parthenope would become hysterical every time the subject of nursing was mentioned.[20]

Parthenope had been ill while her sister was abroad, and Mrs Nightingale thought she was partly upset because she missed Florence. Florence herself had always thought that she and her sister ought to have a better relationship. At 10 years old, she wrote a letter to Parthenope saying: 'I think of you, pray let us love one another more than we have done. Mama wishes it particularly, it is the will of God, and it will comfort us in our trials through life. Goodbye.'[21] That last 'Goodbye' sounds awkward. 'Yours affectionately' was Florence's more usual way of signing her letters.

But their relationship varied between affection and resentment on both sides, and continued, though they were now unmarried adults, still living in their parental homes. 'What is to become of me?' wrote Florence in one of her private notes. 'I can hardly open my mouth without giving my dear Parthe vexation – everything I say or do is a subject of annoyance to her.'[22] She didn't say what she said or did to vex her sister, but there was obviously irritation on her side too.

Their mother seems to have supported Parthenope, who was often ill and more compliant. Florence she found strong-willed and difficult. Many years later, in her 'Notes on the family', Florence recalled:

> *When I was thirty I had an adult evening school for factory girls, which was, on the whole, the most satisfactory thing I ever did. My sister went into hysterics because I attended this. My mother requested me to abstain for six months from doing anything my sister disliked and to give up for that time entirely for her. To this I acceded.*[23]

Parthenope was then 31. It sounds extraordinary that Mrs Nightingale should require Florence to give up her adult evening-school classes because they were so distressing to her older sister. Apparently Florence was a lively teacher, and her students would turn up after a tiring day at work to be re-energised and stimulated by her lessons. No wonder Florence confessed, in another private note:

> *Oh weary days. On evenings that seemed never to end – for how many long years I have watched that drawing room clock & thought it would never reach the ten & for 20 or so more years to do this.*[24]

When the six months were over, Florence resumed contact with her supportive friends. Mrs Nightingale decided that she and Parthenope would visit the spa at Carlsbad so that Parthenope could take the water cure. Reluctantly, she also allowed Florence to spend three months at Kaiserswerth. From references in a letter that Florence sent her, it seems that Mrs Nightingale paid a quick visit to Kaiserswerth herself.

How far did all these efforts help Parthenope? 'When I went to Kaiserswerth the second time for three months,' wrote Florence, 'being then thirty-one, my sister threw my bracelets, which I had offered her to wear, in my face. The scene which followed was so violent that I fainted.'[25] Soon after, Parthenope suffered an emotional breakdown. She was put in the care of Sir James Clark, physician to Queen Victoria, who diagnosed a hysterical condition and advised Florence to stay away from her sister because her presence aggravated it.[26] It sounds as though it required this intelligent doctor to free Florence from the idea that she must sacrifice all her aspirations to take care of her sister.

It was during these turbulent years of family conflicts that Florence wrote the work that she eventually called *Cassandra*. Cassandra was the daughter of King Priam of Troy, whose unhappy prophesies were disbelieved but turned out to be correct, and she was martyred. The work was privately published. Just as Elizabeth's *My Diary* gives a clear account of her development as a mother, so Florence's work, written between 1850 and 1853, provides a vivid picture of how frustrated and trapped she felt. Like

My Diary, Cassandra was published long after its author's death. They are both about the same length, and both were written when each writer felt least sure of herself.

My Diary and *Cassandra* represent the two sides of the 'grand quarrel' that occurred at Lea Hurst. Both are original, thoughtful works. So what does *Cassandra* tell us?

In her daily life, Florence blamed herself for not being more content with all she had. Her mother invited intelligent and gifted guests to Lea Hurst and Embley. 'But why, oh my God, cannot I be satisfied with the life which satisfies so many people?' her daughter asked herself. 'I am told that the conversation of all these good clever men ought to be enough for me – why am I starving, desperate, diseased upon it?'[27]

Florence usually enjoyed listening to people with particular experiences to share, and who would be ready to listen and reply to her questions. She was eager to learn. Her mother's father, William Smith, had been a long-standing member of parliament, and at one time her father wanted to stand for election too. What Florence must have found difficult was having to entertain and listen politely to some of the 'good clever men' who were less interesting than her father and grandfather, who enjoyed the sound of their own voices and regarded her as a delightful captive audience. She was always afraid that she might start daydreaming in the midst of their monologues. It must have been distressing for a woman of her intelligence to see the endpoint that a speaker was slowly leading towards, and she did sometimes daydream, presumably out of sheer boredom.

Her question, 'But why, oh my God, cannot I be satisfied with the life which satisfies so many people?' sounds like a *cri de coeur*. In *Cassandra*, she voiced her brave and lonely answer. She began:

> *One often comes to be thus wandering alone in the bitterness of life without. It might be that such a one might be tempted to seek an escape in the hope of a more congenial sphere...Such a one longs to replunge into the happy unconscious sleep of the rest*

> *of the race! They slumber in one another's arms – they are not yet awake. To them, evil and suffering are not, for they are not conscious of evil.*[28]

What was the evil that she was able to see? Conventional society, she thought, was made by men to limit the role of women, and women had accepted it on these terms. Now that we have heard the outcry of 20th-century feminists who named 'patriarchy' as the source of women's oppression, Florence's complaint sounds obvious. But her desperate language helps us to see how hard it was, even for such a well-educated 19th-century woman, to draw back the curtain masking male power.

'Why have women passion, intellect, moral activity – these three – and a place in society where *no one* of these three can be exercised?' she demanded.[29] 'Passion, intellect, moral activity – these three have never been satisfied in woman. In this cold and oppressive conventional atmosphere, they cannot be satisfied.'[30] Mothers, she wrote, have forgotten their own dreams, and do not recognise that their daughters have romantic fancies while – Florence imagined – they were playing Schubert, reading the *Review*, or embroidering.

Children are nearer to the passion for life. 'A child will fall on its knees on the gravel walk at the sight of a pink hawthorn in full flower, when it is by itself, to praise God for it.'[31] Was this an early memory of something Florence herself had done? There were hawthorns at Embley. And did she, even as a child, only allow herself to praise God when she knew she was by herself?

Once Florence had grown into a woman and entered upper-class society, she discovered, as she put it in *Cassandra*: 'You are not to talk of anything very interesting, for the essence of society is to prevent any long conversations and all *téte-à-tétes*.'[32] That must have felt like torture for someone as intelligent as herself. She continued: 'Then as to solitary opportunities. Women never have half an hour in all their lives (excepting before or after anybody is up in the house) that they can call their own, without fear of offending or of hurting someone.'[33] For herself, Florence knew the tacit rules. That was why she always made sure she was up well before her family, to meditate or to read hospital reports in secret.

Florence's most bitter accusations were not against men, however. They concerned 'the family'. Yet the family is an abstract concept. Each family is composed of individuals. Florence describes her mother in a private note to herself. Her tone sounds sarcastic – it's hard to be sure – but even so Mrs Nightingale sounds a forceful woman. 'My mother is a genius,' Florence declared. 'She has the Genius of Order, to make a place, to organise a parish, to form Society. She has obtained by her own exertions, the best society in England.'[34] This account of her mother may explain a very perceptive comment about Florence herself by Elizabeth when she visited Lea Hurst. Elizabeth wrote: 'She is so excessively soft and gentle in voice, manner, and movement that one never feels the unbendableness of her character when one is near her.'[35] Appearing to be excessively soft and gentle might have been an effective way of dealing with a 'Genius of Order'!

In *Cassandra*, Florence perceived that the stultifying power exerted by upper-class parents on their children amounted to a system. Even when they were adult, and especially if they were women, the 'children' didn't understand how limited their lives were, and saw no reason to free themselves. Here, the intelligent Florence was a century ahead of her time. Gregory Bateson, who started Family Systems Theory (a method of exploring each family as a self-contained system and looking at the ways in which its members related to one another) in the 1950s, was unlikely to have read *Cassandra,* but came to very similar conclusions about families. Florence's discovery was partly based on what she observed about her own family. But she recognised that it was a fragment of a larger 'system'.

> *The family uses people: not for what they are, not for what they are intended to be, but for what it wants them for – for its own uses. It thinks of them not as what God has made them, but as something which it has arranged that they shall be. If it*

> *wants someone to sit in the drawing-room, that someone is to be supplied by the family, though that member may be destined for science, or for education, or for active superintendence by God, i.e. by the gifts within. This system dooms some minds to incurable infancy, others to silent misery.*[36]

Florence describes herself as silently miserable, and in private notes about her sister she states, more than once: 'Parthe is a child.'[37] So that last sentence of the previous passage sounds as if she was thinking of the two of them. If this passage really is an autobiographical example of a system that she could see, perhaps by 'it', meaning the person who decides how to use family members, Florence was thinking of the 'Genius of Order', Mrs Nightingale.

Years later, she wondered whether there could be a better kind of family. 'Are there parents whose type for their family is that their children shall *attain* power, not submit to theirs?' she asked herself in an essay she wrote on families in 1870.[38] But that was far from her thinking in *Cassandra*. Of the family, she wrote: 'It has *destroyed* the individual life.'[39] Here in *Cassandra* the reader can sense Florence's release of anger. All the italicised words represent her underlinings in the manuscript, and express the power of her feelings.

Florence enjoyed novels, and there are several drawings of her, seated and holding a book. But, in *Cassandra*, she describes her concern that novels distracted women from their dependence on their families.

> *What are novels? What is the secret of the charm of every romance that ever was written? The first thing in a good novel is to place the persons together in circumstances which naturally call out the high feelings and thoughts of the character, which afford food for sympathy between them on these points – romantic events they are called. The second is that the heroine has generally no family ties (almost invariably no mother), or, if she has, these do not interfere with her entire independence.*[40]

She meant that a woman reader might identify with the heroine who had no family ties. She could forget how tightly she herself was bound to her family, and especially to an interfering mother. Through fiction, a woman would be soothed into enjoying the vicarious experience of being independent, rather than striving to be independent in reality.

What, then, about marriage? Could a woman find freedom from the constraints of her birth family by marrying? Florence had thought deeply about this. She finally rejected the attractive Richard Monckton Milnes, who had spent nine years courting her. She found it hard to explain, in *Cassandra*, her objections to marriage, perhaps because she hadn't tried it. 'That man and woman have an equality of duties and rights is accepted by woman even less than by man,' was the awkward way she started. Then, with more certainty: 'Behind *his* destiny woman must annihilate herself, must be only his complement. A woman dedicates herself to the vocation of her husband; she fills up and performs the subordinate parts of it.'[41] She must renounce any vocation of her own, which 'does not much signify; she has none to renounce.'[42]

Cassandra begins with one [clearly Florence herself] who 'has wakened too early, has risen up too soon.' Near the end, the writer cries: 'Awake, ye women, all ye that sleep, awake!' And what should these women do, once they are woken? 'The time is come when women must do something more than the "domestic hearth", which means nursing infants, keeping a pretty house, having a good dinner, and an entertaining party.'[43]

And then? 'The next Christ will perhaps be a female Christ.'[44] A bold thought, though Florence said she had heard inmates of Bedlam claiming to be Christ. She didn't say if any of them were women. She admitted that she could hardly imagine any woman being a female Christ. But perhaps, in her daydreams, she had experimented with the possibility for herself.

The seventh and short last section of *Cassandra* begins abruptly: 'The dying woman to her mourners: – "Oh! if you knew how gladly I leave this life".' She says her death (perhaps she meant a symbolic one) took place some years ago, not the death which is about to happen now. Then follows a paragraph that must have meant a lot to Florence, because she repeated parts of it in other contexts.

> *My people were like children playing on the shore of the eighteenth century. I was their hobby-horse, their plaything; and they drove me to and fro, dear souls! Never weary of the play themselves, till I, who had grown to woman's estate, and to the ideas of the nineteenth century, lay down exhausted, my mind closed to hope, my heart to strength.*
> *Free – free – oh! divine freedom, art thou come at last? Welcome, beautiful death!*[45]

Sometimes, a longing for death can be strongest when a person faces an impasse and cannot see any way forward. It is then not the whole person that needs to die, but a way of life. Florence had lived, until about 1850, in the belief that she should submit to the will of God, to her mother, and to the will of Parthenope. She felt that she had heard God's call but was in too great a state of sin for God to entrust her with divine work.

At this point she did not die, but started to change.

Chapter 6

Nightingale: 'No one will act but me'

Nightingale seems to have reached a nadir of misery and depression when she was 30. In December 1850, she wrote:

> *There is not a single night that I do not lie down in my bed, wishing that I may leave it no more. Unconsciousness is all that I desire. I remain in bed for as late as I can, for what have I to wake for?*[1]

Friends took her abroad, to Italy, Egypt and Greece, where she picked up Athena the owlet, to cheer her. But her real recovery was hers alone. She decided to take charge of her life, not dramatically, but by taking small steps that would not distress her family. Slowly, she discovered that she could and must build her own life. Rather than wait for a change of circumstances, she decided to be more active. She wrote:

> *Let me honestly & with simplicity of purpose set to work, not to complain, but to find the means to live. I must take some things, as few as I can to enable me to live. I must take them, they will not be given me – take them in a true spirit of doing thy will – not snatching them for my own will... No one will act but me.*[2]

There wasn't a great deal that she could change, but she set herself some rules to structure her day at home, and that helped her to feel more in control of her life. 'To preserve myself in a healthy state or at least a healthier state – my Holy Ghost tells me to do three things,' she wrote on Whit Sunday 1851. The second of the three steps was simple. Instead of lying in bed 'for as late as I can', she resolved 'to keep to my hour & a half's steady thinking before breakfast. Without this, I am utterly lost – with this, I think I could keep myself alive – thro' the day.'[3]

In a letter to the Catholic archbishop Henry Manning, she confided that her sister had been diagnosed with a brain disease, but that her parents were continuing their lives unchanged.

> *They* [her parents] *are like children playing on the shore of the eighteenth century. Ah! Don't laugh... Under these circumstances, I have but one course to pursue. No one will act but me... I believe I shall go for the present to the duty nearest at hand, to nurse a sick aunt, and wait to see what I can find out to be God's work for me.*[4]

Mrs Nightingale held the conventional belief that an unmarried woman should continue to live with her parents. It would disgrace the family if Florence left home at all, and even more so to train as a nurse. In her mother's view, she was needed at home, and Mrs Nightingale would often say: 'I can't spare you.' Parthenope had suggested all kinds of projects that Florence could do locally, such as running a nursing home near Lea Hurst or Embley. Parthenope would get upset when her sister did not pursue these projects. Finally, in January 1853, Florence wrote a loving letter to her sister, but stated firmly that she couldn't do everything that Parthenope wanted of her.

> *I cannot, during the year's rounds, go the way which (for my sake, I know) you have wished. There have been times when, for your dear sake, I have tried to stifle the thoughts which I feel ingrained in my nature. But, if that may not be, I hope that something better shall be. If I ask your blessing on a part of my time for my absence, I hope to be all the happier.*[5]

With this letter, Florence seemed to release herself from years of feeling guilty that anything she really wanted would upset Parthenope – and that Parthenope must not be upset. She didn't waver, even though Parthenope certainly was upset when her sister was appointed superintendent of the Harley Street Hospital in London.

> *My sister said something to the effect that she could never pass the threshold* [of the Harley Street hospital]. *And though she did pass the threshold, more than once, the first time she ever came was to go almost into hysterics. She hated the place and treated me like a criminal for taking it. And I felt like one.*[6]

'And I felt like one.' Clearly Florence longed for her sister's approval as she did for her mother's. However, once she was appointed by the British government, Parthenope decided that nursing must be worth doing after all. When Elizabeth visited, she was struck by how much Parthenope was doing to support her sister. 'She is devoted – her sense of existence is lost in Florence's,' Elizabeth observed. 'I never saw such adoring love. To set F. at liberty to do her great work, Parthe has annihilated herself.'[7]

But Elizabeth might not have known that this support was very recent. It was a strange reversal. Before her appointment as superintendent of the hospital, it was Florence who was expected to 'annihilate' herself on behalf of her ill sister.

However, Elizabeth didn't collude with the family comparison of the two sisters. She perceived, as many did not, that Parthenope had an identity of her own. She mentioned it briefly: 'Parthe is plain, clever and *apparently* nothing out of the common way as to character; but she *is* for all that.'[8] Time would prove Elizabeth right. Eventually Sir Harry Verney, from the venerable Verney family, proposed to Parthenope. As Lady Verney, rather than the ailing older Nightingale daughter, Parthenope flourished. She catalogued the Verney papers and researched the family history. She also published stories, articles, and five novels. She became ill again as she aged, but that didn't curb her creativity.

This change seems to confirm the power of Fanny Nightingale, as a mother, to define the identities of a pair of siblings: one 'easy', the other 'difficult'. It's a common pattern, and there is no doubt that the strong-willed Mrs Nightingale did this. The usual dynamic is for the 'difficult' one to feel rejected, while the 'easy' one is afraid to lose her or his safe identity as the preferred sibling. Both siblings often feel trapped in their contrasting roles, not just as children, but long into adulthood. Thanks to Elizabeth's perception, and Sir Harry Verney's proposal, there is plenty of evidence that Parthenope became more than her mother's older daughter, and Florence's sister. She developed into an individual person with special talents. Whether Florence ever felt liberated from her identity as 'difficult' is not clear.

One skill that Florence learned from her mother was an understanding of how to maintain a network of influential contacts. Her friends knew that she wanted to practise nursing, and kept her informed about hospitals. Mrs Nightingale was a very efficient organiser, and Florence found that she was good at planning and organising too. From about 1850 on, she discovered that if she set plans in motion without telling her parents, it was hard for them to stop her, however much they disapproved of what she was doing.

She learned a little about nursing from her stays at Kaiserswerth in Germany, and she also went to Paris to learn from the Catholic Sisters of Charity. Her parents weren't keen on her associating with the Catholic Church. However, she seems to have learned a great deal of her nursing from doing it herself. She enjoyed paying attention to detail, and wanted to become familiar with every aspect of patient care. Had she not taken the initiative in getting some training and good experience, she wouldn't have been able to accept the offer to lead a team of assorted nurses to care for the wounded in the Crimean War. Her life, and the lives of many British soldiers, would have been very different.

Florence had a good friend, Elizabeth Herbert, who was on the Ladies' Committee of a new but not yet opened hospital in Harley

Street, London: the Institution for the Care of Sick Gentlewomen in Distressed Circumstances. Elizabeth (Herbert) thought the hospital sounded just right for her friend Florence. In April 1853, she recommended to Lady Charlotte Canning, the Chair of the Hospital Committee, that Florence be appointed as its superintendent. Lady Canning interviewed Florence and was impressed by her. But Florence still needed her parents' consent. Her mother opposed her daughter's appointment. However, even Mrs Nightingale could see that there were several advantages. The ladies on the Committee were all socially respectable. The hospital was neither in Germany nor in France, but in London. Besides, as one biographer put it, 'It was very tiresome to have Flo at home, treating the drawing-room at Embley as if it were the wilderness of Sinai.'[9] In the end, it was Mr Nightingale who took decisive action. He was a peace-loving man and the atmosphere at home was far from peaceful. He gave his own consent to his daughter's appointment, telling her that he would get her mother's agreement as well. He also promised Florence an allowance of £500 a year, as she would receive no salary from the hospital. It was to be paid to her quarterly, which meant £125 every three months. For a wealthy man, this does not sound over-generous. (But then he probably knew Florence's tendency to give away what she had to the poor and needy. An example of this is his wife's observation to Elizabeth on page 72.)

When Lady Canning decided to appoint Florence as superintendent, she could not have guessed at the pent-up energy she had unleashed. Just after the house on Harley Street had been purchased, Lady Canning received a long letter from Florence, who was then in Paris. Here we see the early signs of Florence becoming a brilliant practical organiser. This is the start of several pages of her detailed instructions.

> *The indispensable condition of a home for the purpose we require is 1st that the nurse should never be obliged to quit her 'floor' except for her own dinner & supper, & her patients' dinner & supper – (& even the latter might be avoided by the windlass*

> *we have talked about.) Without a system of this kind, the nurse is converted into a pair of legs for running up and down stairs. She ought to have hot & cold water upon her own floor... the requisites for making poultices, barley water, warming all her medicines, dressings &c &c...*[10]

Many of these ideas would be used in Florence's *Notes on Nursing*, published six years later in 1859, and some of her suggestions are so sensible – the importance of fresh air, for example – that they continue to be a requirement in hospitals today.

Soon the hospital in Harley Street was ready, and Florence became its very active and efficient superintendent. When Elizabeth (Gaskell) visited Lea Hurst, more than a year later, Florence was taking a break from an intense summer of nursing. But she enjoyed telling Elizabeth what she did and Elizabeth, clearly fascinated, recorded the details in a letter to her friend Catherine Winkworth:

> *And now she is head of the Establishment for invalid gentlewomen; nursing continually, and present at every operation. She has a great deal of fun, and is carried along by it, I think. She mimics most capitally the way of talking of some of the poor governesses in the Establishment, with their delight at having a man servant and at having Lady Canning and Lady Monteagle to do this & that for them.*[11]

Elizabeth was impressed at how hard Florence worked:

> *She has been night-nurse and day-nurse – housekeeper (and reduced the household expenses one-third from the previous housekeeper who had been accustomed to economy all her life), mixer-up of medicine, secretary, attended all the operations – and rubbed cold feet perpetually at night – which last I name because they found that one lady jumped out of bed when F.N. was coming round and stood with her feet on the hearthstone in order to have them rubbed.*[12]

The observation that Florence 'attended all the operations...' is interesting. She even attended amputations at the London hospital and later at the Scutari hospitals, which must have been harrowing to observe. But Florence was a scientific student, and wanted precise data as to exactly which amputations were likely to succeed, and therefore the kind of nursing the patients would require afterwards. So she was not horrified, as most ladies of her rank surely would have been, especially by the yelps of pain of British soldiers, but recognised how much she had to learn. She even had the idea of setting up a research station at Scutari so that doctors could visit from Britain and use the hospitals to make their own observations.

No wonder Elizabeth was impressed. Next day, she was 'listening to her [Florence's] letters from Egypt this morning yet not attending to them.' This is interesting because it shows that even Elizabeth's attention could be selective. She seemed to have no difficulty in recalling Mrs Nightingale's anecdotes about Florence, or Florence's account of the cholera outbreak in London during the summer of 1854. 'Only mind!' Elizabeth wrote to another friend, Emily Shaen, 'I felt that I heard them [Florence's speeches that Elizabeth was about to repeat] as being received into the family, not as addressed to myself, so they are rather private.'[13]

Florence had made an agreement with her hospital allowing her to help nurse cholera patients at the nearby Middlesex Hospital. But she undertook to be available and to return quickly if she were needed. She assured the Committee that her first duty was to the hospital that had employed her.

Many of the cholera patients at the Middlesex Hospital were prostitutes. Florence talked to them and had sympathy for them. They didn't have wealthy fathers. They had to earn their keep and, in that respect, were more independent than she was. She wrote to her sister about them:

> *Prostitution is now the most lucrative female employment. You demoralise women by shutting them out of all employments but*

> *governessing and needlework. This is the most fruitful source of female crime. Needlewomen always help themselves out by prostitution and don't blame the ship masters. They ought to be praised, not blamed, for affording women occupation at all.*[14]

This was an original view, and it is very unlikely that Parthenope shared it.

By the time Elizabeth visited, Florence had gained a reputation for being a capable nurse and a very efficient hospital superintendent. She was planning to apply for a similar post as superintendent at St Thomas's Hospital. She mentioned this in Elizabeth's hearing, though she wanted it kept confidential. Her parents and Parthenope were still opposed to her chosen career, although her father was supporting her financially.

In her letter, Elizabeth continued to relate what she heard: 'Speaking of the cholera in the Middlesex Hospital, she [Florence] said, "The prostitutes come in perpetually – poor creatures staggering off their beat! It took worse hold of them than any."'[15] They came from Soho, Broad Street and Oxford Street. 'She herself was up day & night from Friday Sep[tember] 1 afternoon to Sunday afternoon receiving the poor prostitutes as they came in... undressing them – & awfully filthy they were, & putting on turpentine *stupes* all herself to as many as she could manage.'[16]

How much had Florence told her family of what she was doing at the Middlesex Hospital? Her hospital work was a very controversial issue for her mother and sister. But could Florence have felt emboldened by Elizabeth's presence? Her family would hardly have raised their usual loud protestations in front of their literary guest. Besides, we know from a letter by Florence's cousin Hilary Bonham Carter that Florence had enjoyed Elizabeth's novel *Ruth* in 1853, the previous year. (As noted in Chapter 4, *Ruth* is the story of a so-called 'fallen woman': a 15-year-old orphan girl who is seduced, impregnated and abandoned by an upper-class young man.) Florence may also have read *Mary Barton*, in which Elizabeth delicately implies that Mary's Aunt Esther is a prostitute.

'I do so manage to shock people,' Elizabeth wrote.[17] So, listening to Florence, she may have been sympathetic, and perhaps Florence felt sufficiently supported by the author's calm interest to risk being more open than usual about the women she nursed.

How distressing was this to her parents, who had tried to bring up a nice, eligible young lady? In that conversation, Florence did not spare the details. According to Elizabeth, she told her family:

> *'"One poor girl, loathsomely filthy, came in, and was dead in four hours. I held her in my arms and I heard her saying something. I bent down to hear. 'Pray God, that you may never be in the despair I am in at this time.' I said: 'Oh my girl, are you not now more merciful than the God you think you are going to? Yet the real God is far more merciful than any human creature ever was, or can ever imagine.'"'*[18]

Elizabeth, who loved to listen to unusual experiences, continued:

> *Then again, I never heard such capital mimicry as she gave of a poor woman who was brought in one night, when F.N. and a porter were the only people up – every other nurse worn out for the time. Three medical students came up, smoking cigars, and went away. F.N. undressed the woman, who was half tipsy but kept saying, 'You would not think it, ma'am, but a week ago I was in silk and satins; in silk and satins, dancing at Woolwich. Yes! ma'am, for all I am so dirty I am draped in silks and satins sometimes. Real French silks and satins.' This woman was a nurse, earning her five guineas a week with nursing ladies. She got better.*[19]

Those last three words belie the end of the story. It sounds typical of Florence's professional modesty that she didn't add that she was able to nurse the woman back to health. If Florence hadn't stayed on duty when the other nurses were worn out, the woman's story might have ended very differently.

What Mr and Mrs Nightingale made of these revelations is not mentioned. It was exactly the kind of nursing work that they dreaded Florence getting into. There seemed no stopping her. Elizabeth was far too tactful to mention their reactions, though she was sensitive and would have noticed.

And what about Florence herself? She had grown up in a wealthy upper-class family. She was a committed Christian, and almost certainly a virgin. How did she feel about nursing prostitutes? It is difficult to imagine the extremely rigid English class divisions that would have been so familiar to her. Did she have to overcome an initial disgust at undressing and washing 'loathsomely filthy' women? She had a duty as a nurse, and as a Christian, to care for all persons, however dirty and poor. She had rubbed the feet of some of the gentlewomen at the hospital in Harley Street. Was it harder to wash the whole body of a prostitute? She was in a professional role and obviously had enormous energy as a nurse. But there was something more than that too. It wasn't just her sense of duty or her pride in her professional role. She had a profound faith in her connection to individuals of every class and all circumstances, which may explain why even prostitutes felt able to talk to her. In a letter to her father, she wrote:

> *We should consider that the same tie really connects us to every one of our fellows as the tie which connects us to God.*[20]

She seems to have seen prostitutes as desperate women doing their best to survive in an unequal world. This made her very rare among Victorian women. It must have been quite an experience to be nursed, not by rough condemnatory hands, but by hers.

Years later, Florence had to advise on venereal disease in the British Army, so she had to reconsider her views on prostitution. By that time, she was prepared to acknowledge that it was sinful, but still refrained from condemning the women or their individual customers. Instead, she blamed the British Army as an institution for leaving soldiers with time to become bored and idle, and for only intervening when those same soldiers caught a venereal disease. 'No provision was made for the systematic caring for the soldier's *health* but only for his sickness,' she complained in her direct way.[21] She thought the soldiers should be given plenty of honest work to occupy them. Her point was a good one – though she seems to have underrated the strength of young men's sexual energy.

Written to her friend Emily Shaen, Elizabeth's account of Florence's hospital work is followed by a description of their grand quarrel (to be discussed in Chapter 7). Elizabeth concludes:

> *I think I have told you all – even to impressions – but she is really so extraordinary a creature that impressions may be erroneous, and anything like a judgement of her must be presumptuous, and what a letter I have written! Only if you are on the sofa it won't tire you as it might do if you were busy.*[22]

This letter was written when Elizabeth was about to leave Lea Hurst, and when Florence and her nurses were already travelling to huge military hospitals at Scutari. Florence's friends Elizabeth and Sidney Herbert saw this as just as important an opportunity as she did. Florence worried that she would have to break her agreement with the Harley Street hospital. But Elizabeth Herbert reassured her: 'Everyone [on the committee] felt the importance of the work so not a word would be said of any "broken engagement" at Harley Street. This was a "great national work" to which you are called, and it is God's work besides.'[23] Her husband, Sidney Herbert, whose title was Secretary at War to the government, wrote to Florence on 15 October suggesting that she take a party of nurses to Scutari. He said she was 'the one person in England capable of organising and supervising such a scheme.' If she accepted, he told her, 'a prejudice will have been broken through and a precedent established which would multiply the good to all time.'[24]

Despite harrowing reports in the national newspapers, Florence does not seem to have understood how bad things were in Crimea. But she was confident that she could help. She wrote to Elizabeth

Herbert: 'I do not mean to say that I believe the *Times'* accounts, but I do believe that we may be of use to the wounded wretches.' And she wanted to make it clear that she was not merely an upper-class lady of kindly intentions but a professional nurse: 'Would you or someone of my [hospital] committee write to Lady Stanford to say "this is not a lady but a real hospital nurse" of me. And she has had some experience.'[25]

Even when the government appointed Florence and agreed to fund her, she still, as with her hospital appointment, required parental permission to accept the post. As an unmarried woman, then aged 34, she was legally dependent on her father. She wrote: 'My uncle went down this morning, to ask my father & mother's consent.'[26] A letter survives from Mrs Frances Nightingale to Sidney Herbert giving consent to her daughter's appointment.[27]

Florence had mixed feelings about her family's response. She seems to have refused to write 'my' before 'mother' and 'sister'.

> *What have mother and sister ever done for me? They like my glory; they like my pretty things. Is there anything else they like in me? I was the same person who went to Harley St. and who went to the Crimea. There was nothing different except my popularity. Yet the person who went to Harley St. was to be cursed and the other was to be blessed.*[28]

She strove to be charitable, as a good Christian, but understandably set out for Scutari with hurt feelings towards her family.

Chapter 7

Gaskell: 'A grand quarrel'

At first sight, Elizabeth and Florence appear to have many more unusual qualities in common than a major issue to divide them.

The most striking quality, evident in both of them, was a deep humanity. Elizabeth found much to admire in the poor, cold and starving factory workers of Manchester. Florence marvelled at the courage and resilience of the ill-fed ordinary British soldiers in Crimea. Both Elizabeth and Florence wanted the nation to wake up to the enormity of the human suffering that each had witnessed, but that so many of their contemporaries seemed able to ignore.

In the preface to *Mary Barton*, Elizabeth explains her compassion for the poor, women as much as men, on which her novel is based:

> *I bethought me how deep might be the romance in the lives of some of those who elbowed me daily in the busy streets of the town in which I resided. I had always felt a deep sympathy with the care-worn men, who looked as if doomed to struggle through their lives in strange alternations between work and want; tossed to and fro by circumstances, apparently in even a greater degree than other men.*[1]

Elizabeth also wanted to explain the behaviour of profoundly impoverished and disheartened individuals to her readers who might otherwise condemn their behaviour without understanding that they had reasons for resorting to it. So, in *Mary Barton*, she pauses in narrating the story to speak in her own voice. She has just explained that one of the main characters – Mary Barton's father, John, who was jobless, and who had no hope of finding work – was taking opium. Elizabeth then makes a powerful plea to her readers to understand his desperate situation and not judge him harshly for it.

> *But before you blame too harshly this use, or rather abuse* [of opium], *try a hopeless life, with daily cravings of the body for food. Try, not alone being without hope yourself, but seeing all around you reduced to the same despair, arising from the same circumstances; all around you telling (though they use no words or language), by their looks and feeble actions, that they are suffering and sinking under the pressure of want. Would you not be glad to forget life, and its burdens? And opium gives forgetfulness for a time.*[2]

In a similar way, Florence describes the common prejudices against soldiers, which derived from lack of understanding:

> *I have never been able to join in the popular cry about the recklessness, sensuality, helplessness of the soldier. On the contrary I should say (& no woman perhaps has ever seen more of the agricultural and manufacturing classes of England than I have – before I came out here) that I have never seen so teachable & helpful a class as the Army generally... Give them suffering & they will bear it.*[3]

Her utter dedication was felt by the soldiers, and many of them responded to it. One wrote home: 'Before she came, there was cussin and swearin, and after it was holy as a church.'[4] However, not all soldiers were so appreciative; nor was Florence sentimental about them. 'There are one or two scoundrels in every regiment,' she noted, 'and five or six who are not far off from being so.'[5]

When she returned from Scutari, she found that many other women wanted to train as nurses too. She wrote her *Notes on Nursing* to guide them, pointing out simple ways of becoming competent. She advised a nurse to use her senses to observe her sick patients rather than troubling them with excessive questions. A year later, Florence must have realised that many poorer women were acting as nurses within their own families too. She produced a second book, *Notes on Nursing for the Labouring Classes*. 'Every woman is a nurse,' she wrote in her preface. These *Notes* are written in a warm, personal style. And in case a labouring woman feared she might be required to buy expensive medicines, Florence started by emphasising a patient's need for something that came free of charge: fresh air. 'Open the window above, not below,' she advised. And, practical person that she was, she realised that upper windows might have become stuck through lack of use, so she added: 'If your windows do not open above, the sooner they are made to do so the better.'[6] The *Notes* cost 6d (old pence) which wouldn't have been cheap for a labouring family, but perhaps copies were shared.

No one had ever written a simple book on nursing like hers before, and it shows Florence's confidence in the understanding of working people. She was sure they would want to learn. At the Barrack Hospital at Scutari, she was impressed by how many soldiers enjoyed reading, and had set up a library for them.

As children, both Elizabeth and Florence grew up within large extended families, which meant many family gatherings and outings. Both wrote letters filled with news of grandparents, uncles, aunts and cousins. And yet each seemed essentially lonely, keeping a lot to herself.

Both women were serious about their lives. Both believed that every person had a role assigned by God. Florence emphasised this in *Cassandra*. While Elizabeth wrote, at about the same time but independently, to her friend Eliza Fox: 'I do believe we all have some appointed work to do... advancing the Kingdom of God.'[7]

Both firmly held to the importance of truth. Elizabeth was shocked at the outcry of feelings both for and against *Mary Barton* when it was published. She wrote to a friend in January 1849:

> *Some people here are very angry and say the book will do harm; and for a time I have been shaken and sorry; but I have such firm*

> *faith that the earnest expression of anyone's feeling can only do good in the long run, - that God will cause the errors to be temporary, the truth to be eternal, that I try not to mind too much what people say either in blame or praise.*[8]

She had similar problems with *Ruth* and much later with her biography of Charlotte Brontë. It's not surprising that Florence would recognise her courage.

Neither was a conventional Victorian woman. Each valued her independence and did not want to lose it through the usual wifely subservience to a husband. Florence admitted that she had been tempted to marry the brilliant Richard Monckton Milnes. He understood her and admired her greatly. He was sympathetic to Elizabeth too, and wrote to her in praise of *Ruth*. However, the wife he sought would have duties towards him, such as presiding over his breakfast table, for which he was famous. Florence valued his intelligence and understanding, but she knew she would be required to prioritise wifely hostess duties. She could not see how she could fulfil them and yet have time for the training and hospital nursing that she was sure God had planned for her.

Monckton Milnes professed his love for Florence and asked her to marry him. Her parents were delighted with him and considered him an excellent match for her. She was fond of him, and found it hard to justify her reasons for refusing to marry him. When she finally told him of her decision, she herself was surprised at how painful it was, and how often she missed him afterwards. He eventually married another woman, but, as Elizabeth observed and as we shall read in the next chapter, he remained profoundly devoted to Florence. He served for years on the Nightingale Trust, and later his son did too.[9]

Elizabeth had married, but this didn't seem to mean annihilating herself as Florence had described in *Cassandra* (page 82). William Gaskell, a Unitarian minister, believed in the equality of the sexes. Even more unusually, by 19th-century standards, he didn't demand obedience from her. 'I don't believe William would ever have *commanded* me,' she wrote to her friend Eliza Fox.[10]

Besides, Elizabeth didn't believe that a woman's spirit could be totally crushed, even by a conventional marriage. She described the wife of a far more dictatorial husband than her own in her novel *Ruth*. The wife is first presented as obedient to her domineering husband. 'His wife,' Elizabeth wrote, 'was sweet and gentle-looking, but as if she was thoroughly broken into submission.'[11] However, Elizabeth went on to show that even a wife as submissive as this could be roused to anger. Near the end of the novel, the wife, who is also the mother of four children, exclaims: 'I've been a good wife till now. I know I have. I have done all he bid me, ever since we were married. But now I will speak my mind, and say to everybody how cruel he is.'[12] Her husband's threat to punish their eldest son changed her. It gave her the strength to defend her son and to expose her husband.

Mr Gaskell sounds a responsible man. He was a writer and teacher as well as a minister. Through his wife, he got to know Charles Dickens, and Dickens published some of William's work in *Household Words*. As a writer himself, it could well have been William who first recognised his wife's exceptional talent for telling stories. He certainly encouraged her. He never became wealthy, and eventually, from her writing, she earned more than he did. We can see this from a letter she wrote to her American friend Charles Eliot Norton in 1857. She said she thought it would do her husband good to visit America. '& I cd soon earn the passage & travelling money [for William Gaskell],' she wrote confidently.[13] Since she offered to earn the travelling money, she must have known that her husband didn't have it.

Elizabeth eventually earned almost enough to buy her own house, as we shall see in the next chapter. Financially she became independent, which Florence was not. Florence relied on the financial support of her father throughout her life. However, after 1853, she expressed her career independence with great courage, making choices that went entirely against her parents' wishes.

Elizabeth and Florence were both well read. Elizabeth had been sent to a good school as a young girl, while Florence had received superb tuition from her scholarly father. Both women enjoyed novels. It's true that Florence wrote in *Cassandra* how much she objected to women spending time absorbed in romantic stories about independent heroines (page 81). Yet she herself always kept abreast with the latest literature. She read Elizabeth's works soon after they were published. We shall soon see that she even tried writing a novel herself.

Both women enjoyed good conversations and abhorred dull ones. No one could express exasperation at boring conversations better than Florence. From childhood, she kept factual notes of what she learned. She was therefore a brilliant conversationalist herself, and some of her male admirers were in awe of the sheer breadth of her knowledge. But she complained bitterly that she was restricted by her social role, which meant she was not expected to enjoy an exciting conversation but to engage in pointless dialogue. As she protested in *Cassandra*: 'Are they [women] to be employed in sitting in the drawing-room, saying words which may as well not be said, which could be said as well if *they* were not there?'[14] As for herself:

> *I can pursue a connected conversation, or I can be silent; but to drop a remark, as it is called, every two minutes, how wearisome it is! It is impossible to pursue the current of one's own thoughts because one must keep oneself ever on the alert 'to say something;' and it is impossible to say what one is thinking because the essence of a remark is not to be a thought, but an impression.*[15]

Elizabeth wasn't required to sit in an upper-class drawing-room, listening to such conversations. Usually, she listened either with friendly interest, or a sense of humour. She had a wonderful ear for conversation, and must have been listening for little details of pronunciation together with technical terms which she reproduced so brilliantly in her writing. Among her friends, she sounds a lively conversationalist. One friend, Susanna Winkworth, described her vividly:

> *When you were with her* [Elizabeth Gaskell] *you felt as if you had twice the life in you that you had at ordinary times. All her great intellectual gifts – her quick, keen observation, her marvellous memory, her wealth of imaginative power, her rare and acute instinct, her graceful and racy humour, – were so warmed and brightened by sympathy and feeling, that while actually with her, you were less conscious of her power than of her charms. No one ever came near her in the gift of telling a story. In her hands, the simplest incident – a meeting in the street, or talk with a factory-girl, a country walk, an old family history – became picturesque and vivid and interesting. Her fun, her pathos, her graphic touches, her sympathetic insight, were inimitable.*[16]

Both Elizabeth and Florence were sticklers for detail, far more than most people. Elizabeth collected idiosyncrasies of speech of men and women, and of different classes, of dress, of house furnishings, of customs already antiquated in her day – tiny details that went into her novels, brought scenes to life, and are now of historical interest. She believed that women noticed more than men, and entreated Marianne's future husband to tell her more news about their American friends: 'little details which it is "beneath the dignity of man" to put on paper.'[17] She exclaimed in another letter to the father of a bride: 'Oh! do be a woman, and give me all possible details...'[18] Florence, even as a young child, used to make notes in tiny books of facts and figures that she thought would be useful. At Scutari, she used her notebooks to record exactly what she saw. She tried to discover why strong, well-grown soldiers grew so weak and ill, even under her care. So when she was invited to write a report for the government, she had more than enough data to hand. Her report was a damning one. She went into minute details, in her characteristic passionate style, of the conditions in which soldiers lay in the hospital and barracks, especially describing the shortage and filth of the latrines and how these were emptied by orderlies. She listed the basic medicines lacking, the rags for bandaging, the inadequate food, the rats, and the non-existent washing arrangements.

Certainly a quarrel between the two women wasn't inevitable.

Florence, when roused, liked to argue her case. However, Victorian women of her class avoided quarrelling, especially outside their families. They regarded quarrels as vulgar and unladylike. There were polite ways of backing down. Florence had taught herself to be silent when her mother and sister protested at her wish to train as a nurse. She had endured years of opposition from both of them over this. It seems unlikely that she would have wanted to pick a new quarrel with anyone else.

Elizabeth encountered opposition over her novels, and knew how to defend herself. She would stand her ground, though also resort to typically conventional Victorian, very feminine, de-escalating phrases, such as: 'My dear Sir, I should not "quarrel with you" if I had time; but I should say you had mistaken my meaning in two or three things; but perhaps that was my fault. I am feeling so stupid just now.'[19] So she told her correspondent that he had mistaken her meaning – but perhaps that was her fault. She didn't like people to be annoyed with her, and her antennae were quick to spot tension and to respond in soothing ways.

Her unusual strength was her ability to listen and appreciate several ways of looking at a situation. All her novels demonstrate how sensitively she could do this.

The characteristic Victorian attitude to quarrelling is illustrated in George Eliot's *Middlemarch*. Mary and Rosamund, now two young ladies, have known one another since childhood. They have a private dialogue that ends:

> *'Mary, you are always so violent.'*
> *'And you are always so exasperating.'*
> *'I? What can you blame me for?'*
> *'Oh, blameless people are always the most exasperating. There is the bell—I think we must go down.'*
> *'I did not mean to quarrel,' said Rosamond, putting on her hat.*

> *'Quarrel? Nonsense; we have not quarrelled. If one is not to get into a rage sometimes, what is the good of being friends?'*[20]

George Eliot's Mary didn't want their conversation to be defined as a quarrel. 'To get into a rage' seemed a more acceptable way of putting it.

We are now in a much better position to appreciate the complexity of the 'grand quarrel' between Florence and Elizabeth. Elizabeth described it in a letter dated 27 October 1854. That was six days after Florence had sailed to France on her way to Scutari, with her 38 nurses. Only then did Elizabeth describe it briefly to her friend, Emily Shaen, after writing pages of admiration for Florence. At the end of her account of the quarrel, she added further praise of Florence, and closed the subject by saying: 'I think I have told you all.' She then changed the subject to one of her daughters.

Both women would have come to their quarrel feeling strong in themselves. At this stage, Elizabeth's writing of *North and South* was coming on well. And Florence seems to have felt profound and calm relief that God had remembered her at last, and was giving her the work for which she had spent decades praying. She had a tooth abscess, as Elizabeth noted (page 62), but nothing was going to keep her from her task now.

Elizabeth doesn't say what she might have said or done to provoke Florence's outburst. She defines it as a quarrel, but Florence may have seen it quite differently. She could well have thought that in Elizabeth she had found a rare friend who would see the position of women as being as degrading as she did. After all, when she described her work with prostitutes, Elizabeth hadn't seemed shocked. She was clearly sympathetic, both to the prostitutes and to Florence's wonderful way of nursing them. Besides, Elizabeth obviously had a strong social conscience. She had risked unpopularity with two novels, *Mary Barton* and *Ruth*, which had immediately stirred up her readers' emotions and turned her into a national figure. Florence, too, had defied her family, first by insisting on training and then by working as a professional hospital nurse. Both women were rebels. Florence could appreciate how independent Elizabeth was. But she had only won independence for herself. It's clear from *Cassandra* that Florence believed in a time when all women would be free. Surely Elizabeth would understand and agree with her.

Elizabeth prefaced her account of the quarrel by saying that she was looking forward to reading Florence's letters about Egypt, which Parthenope had copied and edited, and which were soon going to be printed. Then, without starting a new paragraph, she continued:

> *She and I had a grand quarrel one day. She is, I think, too much for institutions, sisterhoods and associations, and she said if she had influence enough not a mother should bring up a child herself; there should be crèches for the rich as well as the poor. If she had twenty children she would send them all to a crèche, seeing, of course, that it was a well managed crèche. That exactly tells of what seems to me the want – but then this want of love for individuals becomes a gift and a very rare one, if one takes it in conjunction with her intense love for the race; her utter unselfishness in serving and ministering.*[21]

It's surprising that they both knew what 'crèches for the poor' were. They were day nurseries where poor mothers could leave their babies, enabling them to go to work. They had only recently been introduced in France, during the 1840s. Florence might have been shown one when she was in Paris, training with the Sisters of Charity in 1853. Reports suggest that they were unsanitary and fatal for many babies. However, Florence realised that it would be different if the crèches were 'well managed'. Years later, she was shocked when she read the statistics of many infant deaths due to their poor management in Paris. But, even talking to Elizabeth, she would have had enough hospital experience already to feel certain that, under her own efficient supervision and insistence on cleanliness, even those babies of poor mothers in crèches would have had a good chance of survival.

This sounds typical of her thinking. She had long believed that the work of a disreputable nurse could be turned into a respectable profession. Now she realised that crèches for the poorest workers could be made respectable too, and adapted to become a useful asset for the wealthy. Time has proved her right on both counts.

Besides, what was the role of a mother, from Florence's perspective? Her own experience had shown that her mother had given Parthenope and herself to wet-nurses, as many mothers of their class did. Her next tasks were to employ and supervise nurses and governesses. And what useful work was she doing in the meantime? Mrs Nightingale ran two large homes, and created exclusive house parties of interesting and eligible men, who she hoped would eventually court her daughters. It sounds a managerial role, more than a personal one, leaving an upper-class mother plenty of time, as Florence seems to have seen it, to develop her individual God-given talents, enabling her to do useful work outside her home. As for the babies and children, wouldn't they enjoy the society of other children in a clean, well-run crèche? Hadn't she been happy visiting her cousins, and mightn't the crèches be just as enjoyable?

As a childless woman of 34, it must have taken self-confidence to suggest this to Elizabeth, 10 years her senior and mother of four daughters. On her side, Elizabeth could see the weakness of Florence's idea. Her primary wish for Marianne was that her little daughter would know that her mother loved her. By the 'want of love for individuals', she meant that Florence simply hadn't considered that individual mothers might have powerful feelings of love for their children – nor how individual children might have similar feelings of love for their mothers. She may not have been told of Florence's very painful relationship with her own mother. By contrast, the mothers and children in Elizabeth's extended family, as it's easy to see from Sophia Holland's diary, were fond of one another and enjoyed spending time together. Elizabeth herself was, all her life, close to her four daughters.

Besides, a mother had a responsibility to understand each individual child, and to make good decisions about their upbringing, as she describes in *My Diary*. How could a mother possibly fulfil these important duties if all her babies were corralled into crèches? Elizabeth does not spell out these thoughts in her letter, perhaps because Florence's idea was so extraordinary for its time. Surely Elizabeth's friend Emily Shaen would not need to hear the counter-arguments. They would be obvious. Instead Elizabeth quickly reverts to her admiration for Florence in 'her utter unselfishness in serving and ministering.' In this way, she skilfully contained their quarrel and did not expect her friend to be more than a surprised reader of what had happened.

It sounds as though Florence and Elizabeth were alone in whatever room their quarrel took place. There are no reports by anyone else who had witnessed it. And Florence voiced an idea that she seems to have revealed *only* to Elizabeth. She didn't mention it in *Cassandra*, nor in her longer philosophical and theological work, *Suggestions for Thought*, which she was writing at the same time, from 1852 on. There she protested at the narrow prison of the typical family, the tyranny exerted by parents, and the enslavement of daughters. She described an upper-class nursery in which bored children were confined, with little stimulation from the maids who were usually sewing rather than taking care of them. But she didn't suggest that they should be in crèches. Instead, her ultimate message was positive: 'We want a family which will really love and work together in sympathy, and efficiently.'

Florence's idea of communal crèches for the rich sounds original. Yet new ideas, apparently original, don't usually arise from nowhere. They can usually be traced back to a combination of earlier sources. Was Florence remembering some passages in Plato's *Republic*? Her idea bears some significant similarities. She mentioned the *Republic* in *Suggestions for Thought*. Twenty years later, she challenged the translation of Plato's complete works by the Professor of Greek and Master of Balliol College, Oxford, Benjamin Jowett. He was impressed by her line-by-line comments and told her he was using nearly all her suggestions. 'You are the best critic I have ever had,' he told her. The question is whether she had read the *Republic* before 1854 when she quarrelled with Elizabeth.

It would be surprising if she hadn't. She and Parthenope had received a wonderful education from their father, a graduate of Trinity College, Cambridge. He was a Unitarian and so, like the Unitarian members of Elizabeth's family, he thought girls should receive a good education on a par with that of boys. He was keen to tutor his daughters in ancient Greek and Roman classics. He must have begun early because, at a mere seven years old, Florence wrote to her father in fluent French: 'Cher Papa... J'ai oublié tous mon Latin.'[22] Years later, she recalled:

> *When I was ten, my mother would have no more governesses and my father took us* [herself and Parthenope] *in hand. He taught me* [sic: Parthenope was definitely there too] *Latin and Greek and mathematics and whatever he knew himself. I had the most enormous desire of acquiring – for some seven years of my life, I thought of little else but the cultivation of my intellect.*[23]

Her mother was evidently the decisive force in the family. But through education, father and younger daughter drew close. He was impressed by the depth of her thinking. He taught her ancient Greek and, aged 16, Florence translated Homer. They were both interested in politics, so works by Plato and Aristotle were obvious texts to study. It's likely that they would have read the *Republic* in the original Greek together when Florence was in her teens. In Book V, there is a short discussion about the potential of women. Plato's radical plan to equalise the roles of men and women seems to have caught her attention. When she refers to the *Republic* in *Suggestions for Thought*,[24] she sounds familiar with it.

The *Republic* is an account of an ideal city state, based on rational principles. Plato was concerned with political justice, and with the training needed for special 'guardians' to administer it. At the start of Book V, he questioned whether the ideal state should be run entirely by men. After a discussion, he concluded: 'Then there is no pursuit of the administration of a state that belongs to a woman because she is a woman or to a man because he is a man. But the natural capacities are distributed alike among both creatures [men and women]... for all the woman is weaker than the man.'

He observed that women prided themselves on inferior pursuits, 'weaving, and the watching of pancakes and the boiling pot...'[25] Though he had no doubt that women were the weaker sex, he thought they were capable of doing work of greater social value. This was similar to the view that Florence was to express so passionately in *Cassandra*.

Her idea that women were destined for different kinds of work echoes Plato. Plato believed that each woman had her individual talents: 'one woman has the nature of a physician and another not, and one is by nature musical, and another unmusical... one woman is naturally athletic and warlike and another unwarlike and averse to gymnastics... And again, one a lover, another a hater, of wisdom.' All this was leading to Plato's essential conclusion: 'Then it is likewise true that one woman has the qualities of a guardian and another not.'[26] So Plato's view was that a woman's abilities were not to be encouraged for her individual and personal benefit. She was to use them to serve the common good, embodied in the Republic. The best women, together with the best men, were to be its guardians.

Florence, too, thought women had individual gifts, as we have seen in *Cassandra*, but for her it was a religious perception. She thought God had designed women to serve their creator according to their different gifts. But this sacred design was thwarted because women were forced into virtual servitude by their families. As she put it: 'If it [the family] wants someone [not anyone, but a woman, as she made very clear in *Cassandra*] to sit in the drawing-room, *that* someone is to be supplied by the family, though that member may be destined for science, or for education, or for active superintendence by God, *i.e.* by the gifts within.'[27] Sitting for hours in the family drawing-room to make polite conversation with visitors was, she believed, no way to employ God's gifts.

Like Plato, Florence believed that a woman could and should engage in work beyond her private home. In the public domain, a woman would be able to do useful work for her society. But how could she, if she was an upper or middle-class woman? Her mother, Florence said, would claim that she was 'needed' at home, and especially if she had a baby to care for. It was Plato who suggested a radical solution to enable mothers to work outside the home. He conceived of the Republic as a commune. No one was to have individual property. So a mother could not 'own' her baby. Instead, the Republic's excellent guardians were to organise a few nurses to care for all the babies together in one communal nursery. The babies were to be breastfed, but by any one of a pool of lactating women, not necessarily their mothers. This would release all women to work alongside men, to train as guardians, or to do whatever work their natures had designed for them.

Plato believed in 'good' people marrying one another, and 'inferior' people marrying those like themselves. This was to have a significant outcome.

> *The offspring of the good, I suppose, they* [the guardians of the city] *will take to the pen or crèche, to certain nurses who live apart in a quarter of the city, but the offspring of the inferior, and any of those other sort who are born defective, they will properly dispose of in secret, so that no one will know what has become of them.*[28]

Florence would surely have been curious about part of Plato's plan. Would it be a good idea to appoint a few nurses to care for a crèche of babies? Plato thought that would enable mothers to become guardians, or to do other kinds of useful work. It sounds remarkably like Florence's own justification for crèches. What a simple way that would be to free up all mothers! Plato's plan, however, went further. He would have almost eradicated motherhood. He thought women were necessary in order to bear and give birth to babies. But after that, he intended them to be detached from their newborns by preventing each mother from knowing which baby was hers, and each child from identifying his or her parents. Parenting was to be totally communal. Many years later, when she was helping the classicist Benjamin Jowett to translate the *Republic*, Florence dismissed this idea briskly: 'It is all such nonsense,' she wrote.[29]

She was a critical reader, certainly not in awe of Plato. As an experienced nurse, she pointed out to Jowett that there would be no need for the guardians of the Republic to dispose of 'inferior' babies in secret, 'for they would have died of themselves.'[30] Statistics of the deaths of babies in crèches appalled her. 'It *is* infanticide putting children out to nurse,' she concluded. But, that aside, she would have been horrified by Plato's disregard for an 'inferior' or 'defective' child and his assumption that the Republic must secretly dispose of them. Every child, she believed, had been created by God to live.

Why didn't Florence take her unusual idea further? She must have realised that, even if every mother put her baby into a crèche (however clean and efficiently managed), those mothers would need to be educated and trained before they could do the useful work which she was sure God had destined for them. No institutes existed at that time in England for the further education and training of women. Florence had been resourceful, working against family opposition. She visited hospitals whenever she could, and taught herself how to be a good nurse. But she must have hoped that the very first step towards compelling women to fulfil their God-given destinies would be to liberate *every* mother from the automatic obligation to care for her baby. That would open up the question of what else these liberated mothers were to do. In Victorian England – what a revolutionary idea!

Elizabeth, for her part, was obviously startled at Florence's proposal. How then did she take it? It took her nearly a week to describe it in a letter to one of her closest friends. However, she does not reveal either what she said in reply or how she felt. As the expression goes, 'It takes two to quarrel', and it seems very unlikely that Elizabeth, 10 years older, with four daughters, and 20 years' experience of being a mother, could have listened to this extraordinary idea in total silence. It is much more probable that she would have given Florence a civil but spirited reply. And how would Florence have responded to that?

We will get indications of what must have happened from their subsequent communications with one another. But Elizabeth was right to call it a '*grand* quarrel'. Both women held profound and well-considered beliefs. Both had struggled to live by them. Now both found them challenged, and neither seemed to understand the reasons behind the other's view. Without more time to understand one another, it was impossible to take their difference further.

So, if Florence had hoped for an ally in her conviction that women were wasting their lives, being confined to marriage and motherhood, she would have been disappointed. She wouldn't have had have time to pursue the conversation further as she had meetings to attend in London and much to prepare. Elizabeth for her part must surely have felt deeply hurt. She admired Florence very much, so to quarrel with her and to be unable to discuss it further would have pained her.

More than two years later, after the Crimean War, Florence contacted Elizabeth, and Elizabeth replied. As we shall see, they don't seem to have had any direct contact with one another before then. They respected one another, especially so in Elizabeth's case. They were able to cooperate together over charitable works. But they did not become close and never resolved their difference.

Chapter 8

Gaskell: 'Or will you snub me?'

Elizabeth and Florence were in total disagreement on one issue, and they now had to go their separate ways, but they continued to think of one another.

Elizabeth was left behind at Lea Hurst while the Nightingale family rushed to London to support Florence. She was preparing to take her nurses on the boat to France and then on to Turkey. Elizabeth longed to hear more so she wrote to Parthenope with requests for information at intervals throughout the Crimean War. The first time was on her way home to Manchester, a few days after she had left Lea Hurst:

> *I do so want to hear about you all. I know I have no right from recent acquaintanceship to expect to hear at such a time as this; so I don't come as a claimant, but only as a beggar... I pick up all the scraps I can out of newspapers; but I think they only whet my hunger;...*[1]

Florence remembered Elizabeth too. As a full-time nurse at Scutari, she had discovered a genuine need for novels. She asked for Elizabeth's *North and South* in particular. 'It rests me,' she wrote. She probably meant that a good novel distracted her briefly from all the urgent work she needed to do. This must have felt quite different from reading novels to fill time at home in the evenings. She wrote to her family from Scutari in April 1855:

> *Do send me this year's numbers of* Household Words. *I want to read* North and South. *It rests me. No one sends us any but such old numbers. You sent us up to December and I read them.*[2]

A month later, Elizabeth, longing for more news, wrote a quick note to Parthenope:

> *Only best wishes and kindest regards. I have time for no more. But I often think of you & her, & you all. You'll let me have one line to say how she is.*[3]

In May 1855, Florence became seriously ill and nearly died. She called her illness 'Crimean Fever' but it has now been identified as brucellosis (a bacterial infection from unpasteurised milk and cheese. One of the commonest symptoms is a recurrent fever.)[4] She survived, but the fever recurred many times when she was back in England. However, by August 1855 she was up and active again, as we can see from her letter to her close friends Charles and Selena Bracebridge. Near the end of a long letter, Florence wrote:

> *The thing I would like best if you would send me would be a good novel – not fashionable like Mrs Gaskell's* North and South, *which you also might send us in its whole edition (I have read it in* Household Words*) for the reading room. When I lie down, which I never do, I think of all the things to be done, and they start me up again. If I had a good novel, perhaps I should not think of them.*[5]

At that time, Florence didn't realise that Elizabeth had expanded the ending of *North and South* in the complete two-volume edition. It was less rushed, and perhaps Florence would have considered this version 'good' too. The 'reading room' was a library she had helped to set up for wounded soldiers. She was impressed at how many of them enjoyed reading.

She herself had, as she said, a lot to think about. The four hospitals at Scutari were in chaos. The doctors there resented any interference from mere nurses, so it was frustrating for someone as efficient as she was to hold back. A few weeks after arriving, she vented some of her fury about the medical practitioners back home:

> *But oh! You gentlemen of England who sit at home in all the well-earned satisfaction of your successful cases can have little idea from reading all the newspapers of the horror and misery* [at Scutari], *of operating on all these dying and exhausted men – a London hospital is a garden of flowers to it.*[6]

With energy that astonished those who saw her, she knelt on filthy floors, amid all the flies, scurrying rats and appalling smells, and bound soldiers' wounds. She had a complete disregard for contagion, and nursed those who were ill from typhus and cholera (which was considered contagious then, but has since been identified as being caused by sufferers drinking contaminated water), often staying with the very ill until they died. She was also present at the most serious amputations. She did her best to order clean bedding, clothes, and wholesome food. A report stated: 'Real milk was provided for the patients in some of the hospitals by Miss Nightingale.'[7] And indeed she became known as 'the lady with the lamp' because she liked to walk through the hospital wards when it was quiet at night, and very peaceful. She would listen to the patients who needed practical nursing and comfort, until she could convince herself that she had done everything possible.

She couldn't reach everyone. The Barrack Hospital at Scutari was enormous, 'little less than four miles of ground occupied in lines of beds,' wrote Lord Sidney Godolphin Osborne, who went to help in 1855.[8] He was impressed by Florence. 'Her general demeanour is quiet and rather reserved; still I am much mistaken if she is not gifted with a very lively sense of the ridiculous,' he wrote.[9] There must have been plenty to ridicule in the mismatch between the reality of Scutari and the assumptions made about it in London.

Stories abounded of Florence's gentleness and wonderful ability to help the very ill. Lady Augusta Stanley provided a characteristic example. She reported that:

> *A Captain Sandby, just come back* [from Scutari] *says five wounded men were brought to the hospital in such a state of*

> *exhaustion the doctor gave them up; Miss Nightingale undertook them, washed their wounds, fed them, watched them through the night and brought them round. The three head medical officers write in the strongest terms of what she had done.*[10]

This was exactly the kind of information that Elizabeth wanted. She begged Parthenope for news in a letter dated early August 1855: 'Every scrap & crumb is more than welcome.'[11] and in October 1855: 'Please ask me again, sometime to Lea Hurst... My kind regards to Mr and Mrs Nightingale. Please thank them from me. And when you have time a crumb from Scutari.'[12]

In January 1856, Elizabeth wrote to Parthenope, this time with information about a meeting she had attended in Manchester.

> *When some of the mills 'loose' their workpeople, plenty of grimy hands came in, all ready to cheer and applaud their heroine – for they feel her* [Nightingale] *as theirs, their brother's nurse, their dead friend's friend – in a way which they don't know how to express. 'You benevolent ladies! Why you women all play at benevolence – Look at Florence Nightingale – there's a woman for you!'*[13]

In the same letter, Elizabeth mentioned Florence's friend and one-time suitor, Richard Monckton Milnes. He was older, had married, and was well known (though not to Florence) as a homosexual. By then, he had lost his youthful looks. He too spoke at that same meeting. Elizabeth described him to Parthenope:

> *Dear Mr Milnes! His speech warmed my heart the most. He evidently forgot us all, in bringing up before himself pictures of former days; of Florence Nightingale as a girl in her father's house, – of his early knowledge of her, &c. His face grew quite pale, & you forgot that fat in the features – the eyes fixed on by-gone scenes, not on all our poor upturned faces.*[14]

Elizabeth was not alone in wanting to hear more about Florence. People in England, whether wealthy or poor, were fascinated by stories of what she was doing for the wounded soldiers at the Barrack Hospital, and Elizabeth's account reflects this.

In August 1856, while Florence was returning to England with her aunt Mai, as unobtrusively as possible (she had refused an invitation to return on a splendid man-of-war ship), Elizabeth replied to a letter from Parthenope:

> *I did like your letter. I was so glad to get it, you can not think, dear Miss* [Parthenope] *Nightingale. Every scrap you can ever tell me about her is most valuable to my heart. God bless you both.*[15]

'Both,' Elizabeth ended her letter. She probably sensed Parthenope's readiness to compare herself unfavourably with her gifted sister. Elizabeth, with her usual sensitivity, was keen to demonstrate to Parthenope that she was interested in her as well as in her sister.

Florence arrived back in England on 7 August 1856. She travelled to London with her favourite aunt, took a train to Derby, and arrived on foot at Lea Hurst in the late evening. By this time she was a national heroine. There were stories in *The Times* about the lady with the lamp who tended wounded soldiers while asking nothing for herself.[17] Queen Victoria invited her to Balmoral and was impressed by her. Yet Florence, who had daydreamed for years about accomplishing heroic deeds for which she would be widely acclaimed, while berating herself for her 'sinful' daydreaming habit, found that in reality she didn't at all relish being a much-admired heroine.

Elizabeth's own life was busy. She, too, had found fame difficult. *Mary Barton* was published anonymously, but its authorship was soon discovered, and people pointed her out in the street. 'Oh dear!' she wrote. 'I wish poor Mary Barton could be annihilated this next month; and then I might go where I liked, & do & see what I liked naturally and simply.'[18]

Patrick Brontë asked her to write a biography of his daughter Charlotte, who had died in March 1855. Elizabeth had never attempted a biography before. She did extensive research, visiting places where Charlotte had lived, discovering letters written by and about her, and interviewing people who remembered her. The finished biography was published in 1857 as *The Life of Charlotte Brontë*, but caused offence to some who remembered her, and Elizabeth, much against her will, had to revise her work. She also continued to write short stories for *Household Words* and other journals.

In December 1858, when she came home from a trip to Germany and France, she discovered she had been sent a packet from Florence Nightingale with a covering letter, dated 1 December 1858.

Little could Elizabeth have known how many other people had received a package with the same contents, together with a personally crafted letter. Florence had put together a brilliant confidential report with the title: *Notes on Matters Affecting the Health, Efficiency and Hospital Administration of the British Army 1858*. She also wrote and included her *Subsidiary Notes as to the Introduction of Female Nursing into Military Hospitals in Peace and War*. The report was commissioned by Lord Panmure, and Florence paid for a number of copies to be printed for private circulation. It ran to 853 pages, and not many people read it. She complained bitterly: 'They have *not* read the *Notes* but they have *talked* about the *Notes*.'[19] Her report included many letters from generals and politicians. But it was her own narrative that was the most impassioned, and her authentic voice comes through from the 1850s to today. She doesn't mask her fury at the inefficiency she saw. She describes in great detail the overcrowding of patients in the hospital buildings and adds, indignantly: 'So that it may safely be said that, treated under a hedge, they would have had more chance of recovery.'[20] Nor does she spare the nurses in her charge: 'All nurses, male and female, should be able to read directions.'[21] 'How is it that the food of the soldier was bad? that he had in Bulgaria sour bread, in the Crimea, biscuit? that he had in Bulgaria bad meat, sometimes goat's flesh, in the Crimea, salt meat?... How was it that fuel was not provided?'[22]

Then, explaining to each recipient that the report was highly confidential (because, although she had sent copies to the War Office and Queen Victoria, she hadn't yet presented it to the House of Commons), she sent at least 14 copies, between October and December 1858, to chief army officers, to members of the House of Lords, and to the Dean of St Paul's Cathedral. Finally, on 30 November and 1 December, she sent copies to two writers. One was Harriet Martineau and the other was Elizabeth Gaskell.[23] Each of these 16 recipients would have got the impression, from the courteous personal letter that Florence enclosed, that he or she was the sole and very special person to have been entrusted with this confidential report.

Why did Florence send her report to Martineau and Gaskell? They were writers, not politicians. But perhaps that was exactly why she chose them.

Several times, when she was at Scutari, she compared the terrible suffering she saw there to the sufferings described by the ancient Greek tragedians, Aeschylus and Sophocles.[24] On another occasion, she was reminded of Shakespeare's lines about English soldiers at the Battle of Agincourt. She wrote that she recognised, in the British soldiers fighting in Crimea, 'the same courage, and unflinching endurance, but the same suffering, the same famine, and far greater mortality.'[25] All this would be worthy of a great novel.

Clearly Florence was considering two writers who were well known for their ability to move people by their accounts of social evils. She herself had experimented with writing a novel before the Crimean War, sometime between 1850 and 1853,[26] but this was never published in novel form. It was a dialogue between a mother and daughter, discussing the predicament of women. It reads more like a tract than a story. Unlike the novels of Gaskell and Dickens, it distinctly lacks humour. It ends with the daughter crying: 'Free, free. Oh!... welcome beautiful death!' as she falls face-down and dies. The penultimate sentence of *Cassandra* was identical.

Now Florence had written a passionate report. But this did not have the national appeal of a novel. She wanted the British reading public to know about the courage and suffering of the brave soldiers who fought in the Crimean War. Martineau and Gaskell had reached their readers in ways that she could not.

To Harriet Martineau, Florence wrote:

> *Dear Madam, I know that you have been interested about our army matters... Therefore it is only for your own private reading that I send it, if you still have time, strength or inclination for this kind of subject. If not, please put it in the fire.*[27]

Martineau was the right person to send the report to. Florence wrote on 30 November, and Martineau's reply is dated 3 December. She wrote:

> *My dear Miss Nightingale, I have waited a day to acknowledge the arrival of the* Report. *It is now before me & I have to thank you, which I do very cordially, for the painful pleasure I foresee I shall have in reading it. I need not say that your wishes as to privacy shall be exactly observed. I suppose they do not preclude any use that I may be able to make of facts in the* Report *– as facts, without citing you or the Report. What I mean is that I still write for the 'Daily News'... & it would be a great benefit to do it again under the enlightenment of your information.*[28]

She wrote six leaders for the *Daily News,* and sent them to Florence to check the facts before publishing them. Florence was very grateful to her: 'All *such* help is most valuable to us.' Later, with more enthusiasm, 'So few people give me that kind of sympathy... so very few.' And a few weeks later she signed a letter to Martineau: 'ever yours overflowingly, Florence Nightingale.'[29]

Meanwhile, Florence had heard nothing from the other writer she had chosen. Martineau had replied almost by return of post. Florence had written to Elizabeth on 1 December 1858 – but

Elizabeth didn't reply until 31 December.

Elizabeth had had up to a month to wonder why Florence had sent her such a confidential document. She had written to Parthenope many times during the war, asking for news. So perhaps she thought Florence had sent her the document to satisfy her curiosity, and enable her to learn more about conditions at Scutari. However, this wasn't the explanation that Florence gave her.

It's worth looking at their exchange closely to see what it reveals about them both.

Florence began her letter: 'Dear Mrs Gaskell, I wonder whether you ever remember me...'[30] So presumably the two women hadn't been in touch with one another for some time. Elizabeth was warmly reassuring: '*Don't* I remember you?' she replied.

She needed to explain why it had taken her so long to reply.

> *My dear Miss Nightingale, I was in Paris, as you would hear when your letter & the 'Confidential Notes & Subsidiary Notes' arrived. I thought you would not care for the mere form of acknowledgement which I could have sent immediately on my coming home: so I waited until I had read something of them.*[31]

Florence's letter continued: 'and whether you ever think of all the army matters which have made up my life for the last four years'.

Elizabeth was keen to respond to this because she had thought a great deal about Florence and the soldiers, in battle and in hospital. But she wanted to preface her response with a misgiving as to how Florence would receive her words.

> *And now may I say what is in my heart: or will you snub me à la Dr Johnson? I don't believe you will, because it is so very true, & moreover I will try not to praise or honour you a bit.*

Curious that she thought Florence might snub her. Florence was sharp in her condemnation of inefficient government ministers and army chiefs. There are many scathing examples in her report.

But Gaskell didn't belong to either category.

Could Elizabeth have been recalling their 'grand quarrel'? Could Elizabeth have protested, there and then, at Florence's complete dismissal of the value of mothers? But Florence had meant what she said. She believed mothers were enslaved to their husbands and children. She was free from those ties and about to fulfil what she believed was the work that God wanted her to do. So had she replied impatiently? Once roused, she could be sharp in defending herself. And could this explain why Elizabeth felt snubbed, and feared being snubbed again?

However, Elizabeth quickly back-tracked, saying that she was sure she wouldn't be snubbed. And she must have heard that Florence didn't like 'praise or honour.' Her assurance that she respected this sounds as if she is soothing any hard feelings that Florence might have had towards her.

With that preface, Elizabeth felt able to explain how much she had thought about Florence's work at Scutari.

> Don't *I remember you? – and* haven't *I thought of you? – & your soldiers & your army matters? Little bits that your sister told me long ago about your soldiers come up in my mind in the dead of night often & often, & one can't be strongly interested in individuals without learning to care for the class to which they belong.*

This might have sounded hopeful to Florence. If a novelist as good as Elizabeth thought about her and the soldiers in the dead of night, might she not want to write about them? Florence's letter continued:

> *I never know whether people can be really interested in our men, can lay aside the British prejudice against 'the soldiers' who have not seen them as I have in their heroic simplicity and unmurmuring patience under suffering the most tedious and harassing.*

She was apparently looking for agreement that there was British prejudice against soldiers, but without suggesting that she believed Elizabeth herself would not have shared it. Elizabeth, however, must have read this sentence differently. Her reply shows that she thought Florence would like to hear that British prejudice against soldiers had diminished.

> *Besides you know I live in the very midst of what was once called the 'Peace party' – (Manchester has really as pretty a fighting spirit as anyone could wish to see, –) and formerly, before the Crimea, I constantly heard the 'army' spoken lightly of, if not positively sneered at – and now all speak with respect of soldiers, – since that winter in the trenches. It is a great change in manner of speaking & thinking, & as good a testimony as I think can be brought to the gradual acknowledgement of the noble qualities called out by the discipline & dangers of a soldier's life.*

Here the two women are surely writing at cross purposes. If Elizabeth was right that the British had changed their attitude towards soldiers, then the position of soldiers would be less tragic than Florence supposed. Soldiers who were tragically misunderstood because of a British lack of understanding would make a much better subject for a novel or story.

Florence had then asked for assurance of confidentiality:

> *May I venture to send you a copy of a 'confidential' report (by me) to the War Office for your own reading only. For it is really "confidential," and must not be seen, please, out of your own family. It is in no sense public property... May I ask you not to mention to anyone that you have this report? I have no right to give away a single copy, the thing not having been presented in the House of Commons.*

Florence was taking a risk in sending her confidential report to Elizabeth. Elizabeth was a sociable woman who travelled, met people, and enjoyed good conversation. How discreet would she be? She might easily mention something from the report by accident, revealing that she had read it. Elizabeth didn't reassure Florence on this point until the end of her letter: 'No one shall see those books but my own family. Nor does anyone know that I have them. God bless you!'

Florence continued her letter:

> *It is an old story now but may interest you, I think, still, not by any means as a literary work, to which it has no pretension, but you, whose interest is so intense for the class from which the soldier still springs, may like to see what was and is the real account of his sufferings, both then and now, both in war and in peace, now up to this present moment...*

It's significant that Florence admitted that her report was not a literary work, and wasn't pretending to be one. This sounds like a hint that there was a place for a genuinely literary work on the subject, and that Elizabeth might be a good person to write it: 'you, whose interest is so intense for the class from which the soldier still springs,' may express the hope that Elizabeth would be moved by the injustice towards soldiers who had suffered so much. It was two-and-a-half years since Florence had returned from Scutari, and she was obviously haunted by the sheer magnitude of the suffering and courage she had witnessed. She wanted it to be widely known.

But Elizabeth could easily have read the first sentence as Florence's apology for asking her to read a work that wasn't up to her own literary standard. She might also have concluded that she had been sent the report because she 'may like to see what was.' Perhaps Florence had learned from her sister how often Elizabeth had begged to know more.

Florence was probably reluctant to ask Elizabeth directly to write something, in case it looked as if she had put her up to it.

Martineau seemed to know what was wanted without being told. But Elizabeth was a modest woman. Besides, she had a profound admiration for Florence. It seems very unlikely that she could have guessed that this dedicated nurse, who had become a national heroine, should want her to write about the brave soldiers. After all, it was Florence who had first-hand experience of them. And besides, Elizabeth was already very busy with her own writing. She had just finished several stories for *Household Words,* and now was working on *Round the Sofa and Other Tales*, which came out in 1859. This, too, would soon be read by Florence.

Elizabeth's letter continued:

> *I read the* Subsidiary Notes *first. It was so interesting I could not leave it. I finished it at one long morning sitting – hardly stirring between breakfast and dinner. I cannot tell you how much I like it, and for such numbers of reasons. First, because you know of a varnish which is as good as or better than black-lead for grates (only I wonder what it is).*

Oh, what a pity that her first response to the *Subsidiary Notes* was to mention the varnish! She probably wanted to show that she had read them with her usual attention to detail, and to create a sisterly rapport with its writer. But this might have been a disappointment to Florence. She didn't build rapports over domestic details.

Elizabeth continued to write about the *Subsidiary Notes:*

> *Next, because of the little sentences of real deep wisdom which from their depth and true foundation may be real helps in every direction and to every person; and for the quiet continual references to God which make the book a holy one.*

Here, she may have been more in sympathy with Florence, who felt she was doing the holy work which God had destined for her, though she had also written with a good deal of anger against those in power who, through their incompetence, had allowed soldiers to suffer. Elizabeth continued:

> *Now all this has nothing to do with your soldiers, but don't think the book thrown away on me, because I have not sooner said that I had no conception what those poor fellows had had to go through till I had read the larger book of notes – One can hardly believe it – much less realise it. The larger book should have been read first; it is both a tougher subject; & or infinitely the most painful.*

So, at last, here was a woman who had read the whole work. Did Florence appreciate this and respond? Perhaps she did, but Lynn McDonald, who edited *The Collected Works of Florence Nightingale* in 16 scholarly volumes, has not included a reply to Elizabeth's letter. So, if there was one, it has yet to be found.

Near the end of her letter, Elizabeth asks:

> *I only wish you could ever tell me what I might or could do to serve you & yr interests. Mind you do, if I ever can. And don't think this letter impertinent, because you don't know how much I have restrained & kept back.*

Evidently Elizabeth still felt nervous of Florence's response to her, because, having written her letter, she feared to be thought 'impertinent'. However, Florence must have remembered her request. She needed all the help she could get for her immense task. Later, she wrote to make several practical requests of Elizabeth, though the first was not until October 1860.

Meanwhile, Florence continued to be interested in Elizabeth's writing. A few months after their exchange of letters, she wrote an undated note to her mother, asking her to send a copy of Elizabeth's *Round the Sofa*, published in March 1859. Florence seems to have read works soon after they were published, so her request probably dates from then.

Since her return from Scutari, Florence was ill intermittently with recurring fevers and other symptoms of brucellosis. When she was ill, she resorted to reading. On 6 September 1859, Elizabeth received a letter from one of Florence's favourite cousins, Hilary Bonham Carter. It's not clear whether Bonham Carter told Florence that she would write, or whether Florence wanted her to do so. The letter reads:

> *Dear Mrs Gaskell, It is a little thing that makes me think of writing to you, and yet a little thing that methinks will give you pleasure. I thought so this morning when Florence said of your* Ruth*: 'It is a beautiful novel and I think I like it better still than when I first read it six years ago.' Further she observed how you had not made Ruth start at once into a hospital nurse but arrive at it after much other nursing that came first.*[32]

In the following year, Florence sent Elizabeth her *Notes on Nursing.*[33] Perhaps she decided to do so because of her admiration for *Ruth*, and the thought that Elizabeth might want to learn more about nursing for a subsequent novel.

Later that year, Florence had obviously recovered and wrote to Elizabeth asking for practical help with a soldiers' home. Elizabeth raised £120 for the cause, and Florence thanked her for her 'magnificent subscriptions.'[34]

Elizabeth continued to write novels. *Sylvia's Lovers* was published in February 1863. She sent Florence a copy. In June, Florence wrote to her father: 'Would you send up my *Sylvia's Lovers* by Mrs Gaskell, which Parthe took to Embley?' 'My' *Sylvia's Lovers*, she wrote – so if Parthenope had not borrowed her sister's copy and left it at Embley, we wouldn't know that Florence was reading it. On 17 August 1863, Elizabeth received a letter of acknowledgement that Florence was pleased to have been sent a copy of *Sylvia's Lovers.*[35]

Elizabeth's warm response is dated 22 August 1863:

> *My dear Miss Nightingale, Nothing could have made me more pleased to think that I had written 'Sylvia' than to know that it*

> *had given you one hour's enjoyment or timely change of thought – Thank you for accepting it so kindly.*[36]

By coincidence, both women moved into new homes in the autumn of 1865. In October, Florence moved to a house in South Street, London, paid for by both her parents. She lived in South Street, though in different houses, until she died in 1910, aged 90 and not in good health, but constantly active.

Elizabeth was not in good health either, and she too was active. She took the bold step of buying her own house in Hampshire. Her husband was committed to his teaching and pastoral work in Manchester and didn't want to move south, whereas she did. She didn't tell him about the house. It was an incredible achievement that she was managing to pay for most of it from her own earnings. 'I bought a house and 4 acres of land,' she explained to Charles Eliot Norton, a friend in America, 'in Hampshire – near Alton – for Mr Gaskell to retire to & for a home for my unmarried daughters... The house is large in a very pretty garden (kitchen flower-gardens & paddock between 3 & 4 acres.'[37]

The Hampshire house needed much work to make it habitable. Elizabeth was concerned about the details, which constantly distracted her from writing. In addition, she was worried about the health of Meta and Julia, two of her daughters, and also understandably anxious about getting behind with her current novel, *Wives and Daughters*, which was again being published in serial form. 'I have been very ill all autumn,' she wrote to Florence Nightingale in December 1864.[38] She didn't complain easily, but, in February 1865, she told George Smith, one of her publishers, that she was 'feeling so far from strong.'[39] Then, to Smith again in April: 'I broke down in Paris, & for the last fortnight could not leave the house till the day I came here [London].'[40] In August, she wrote to her daughter Marianne that she had been ill for three weeks, and that 'I must save all my health and strength for writing.'[41]

Nevertheless, she continued leading an active life. She visited Dieppe in September, which meant turning down several social invitations including one from the Nightingales, '(and this I *did* regret)'[42] she told Marianne. Many of her letters from these months show how often she was 'in a fidget' about many very practical details – about servants, clothes, and much else. It was not surprising that she must have felt exhausted, and exclaimed at the end of a letter to Marianne: 'oh *how* dead I feel!'[43]

Elizabeth returned from Dieppe to her newly bought house, and was there in November with three of her daughters. She said she felt younger and seemed much stronger and in good spirits. So it came as a total shock to all of them on 12 November when, as they were drinking Sunday afternoon tea in the drawing-room, she collapsed mid-sentence from a heart attack, fell into Meta's arms, and died instantly.

She was buried in Knutsford, at the old Unitarian Brook Street Chapel. William and two of her daughters would also be buried there.

News reached Florence a few weeks later. She sounds upset when she mentions it, halfway through a long letter of family news, dated 28 November, and perhaps addressed to Mai, her father's sister: 'Poor Mrs Gaskell! You will be much shocked to hear of her sudden death from apoplexy, but Aunt Julia who arrived at Thomas House the very day after it will tell you the particulars.'[44]

It is interesting to discover that, years after their quarrel, Florence must have had second thoughts about putting all babies, rich as well as poor, into crèches. All her life, she had been interested in statistics, and was impressed by the work of a Belgian statistician, L.A.J. Quetelet. He demonstrated that babies taken from their families survived less well. In her essay on the family, she reflected:

> *It is now commonly observed that, in the poorest labouring family, if one child is taken away and placed by charity in the most carefully managed asylum, the asylum-bred child does not generally turn out so well, even as the rest.*[45]

She went still further. In a complete reversal of her ideas about the power of families that she so angrily expressed in *Cassandra*, and in her quarrel with Elizabeth, she now thought that children were best cared for within their families. She was as adamant about this as she had been earlier when she argued the opposite view to Elizabeth:

> *For children can only be brought up in families. There is a subtle sympathy between the mother and the child which cannot be supplemented by other mothers.*[46]

Florence herself had been brought up by her mother, but Mrs Nightingale had been ill after giving birth to her, and the newborn Florence was wet-nursed. Her father signed a contract with the Italian wet-nurse Umiliana Pistelli.[47] Florence's feelings about this can be seen in a note she wrote, some 50 years later:

> *Then the strange mistake about mothers not to suckle their own children, as if with the greatest care in selecting the nurse we did not know that she could only be a miserable makeshift for the mother. As if God did not know best, had not provided for this, and the mother's milk were not adapted for her own child and no other.*[48]

She was right that the constituents of a mother's breastmilk are adapted precisely for her own child. But if mothers were the best people to suckle and bring up their children, how could they also fulfil their potential in doing the work for which God, she believed, had destined them? This conundrum is still with us and will be taken up in Chapter 10.

Florence thought a mother should be judged not only by her feelings, but also by her actions. In another private note, she drew a damning comparison between a mother and child, between herself and the 18,000 British soldiers that she saw as her 'children' as well as her hospital patients, and finally between her own mother and herself.

> *When we consider what a mother's feeling really is for her child, how flimsy, how unsubstantial it is... But, in reality, for every one of my 18,000 children, for every one of those poor tiresome Harley St creatures, I have expended more feeling & action in a week than my mother has expended for me in 17 years.*[49]

Her sweeping dismissal of a mother's feelings for her child doesn't sound fair. And a nurse's work differs from a mother's, despite some overlap. Yet, in some rare letters and private notes, she confessed to her own feelings that she regarded as maternal for her patients at the Harley Street hospital, soldiers in Crimea, and a few favourite nurses.

It's moving to learn how haunted she felt by the soldiers whose lives she had not been able to save. Safely back in England, she thought of them constantly. In a private note, dated about six months after she had returned from Scutari, she addressed the soldiers in imagination:

> *Oh my poor men, who endured so patiently I feel I have been such a bad mother to you, as to come home & leave you in your Crimean grave. 73 per cent in eight regiments during six months from disease alone – who thinks of that now? But if I could carry any one point which would prevent any part of the recurrence of this our colossal calamity... then I should have been true to the cause of those brave dead.*[50]

And using similar words, in a long letter to Lady Charlotte Canning, chair of the hospital in Harley Street, she wrote: 'Oh my poor men, who died so patiently I feel I have been such a bad mother to you, coming home & leaving you in your Crimean graves, unless truth to your cause can help to teach the lesson which your deaths were meant to teach us.'[51]

Florence certainly strove to tell the truth in her extensive reports. But she seems to have felt permanently guilty that she could never do enough. She knew her own mother had only two daughters and had failed the younger of them. How much worse was it for her to fail thousands of soldiers? No wonder she didn't want to be fêted as the lady with the lamp. She must have felt that she didn't deserve it.

After the war, she never set foot in a hospital again, though she was proactive in setting up the Nightingale Training School for Nurses. She wanted it to be an independent enterprise, run entirely by women, who would train nurses to a high professional standard. All women from the poorest working classes to ladies of high birth would undergo exactly the same disciplined training. It was a bold vision. Nothing like this existed anywhere.

She was often bed-bound with complications from brucellosis. Yet she persuaded her influential friends and government members to visit her. Her immediate concern was the state of the British Army stationed in India. She developed a brilliant understanding of statistics, and was able to present them in an original diagram form to demonstrate the importance of good hygiene. Today, 'statistician' has been added to the Wikipedia entry for her: 'English social reformer, statistician and the founder of modern nursing.'

Through her single-minded determination, Florence promoted reforms and saved the health and lives of British soldiers serving in India. She might have felt guilty about what she hadn't done – but our lives today would be quite different without the work she *did* manage to do.

She died in her sleep in 1910. She wanted her body to be used for medical research, but her wish was overridden. Instead, it was suggested that she be buried in Westminster Abbey as a token of the nation's gratitude for her work. Her parents and sister were long dead by then, but members of her surviving family knew she would not have wanted this. She is buried beside her parents in the churchyard of St Margaret's, East Wellow, near the larger Nightingale house at Embley.[52]

Chapter 9

Nightingale: 'Treat them like reasonable beings'

This penultimate chapter deserves an explanation. It's not central to the main narrative. But I felt I couldn't leave two such brilliant thinkers without discussing some of their major innovations which are often overlooked or misunderstood. For the main narrative, it would make sense to proceed to Chapter 10, and return here later.

Both Florence and Elizabeth discovered that it was possible to reason with vulnerable people. Reason was not the prerogative of the educated. As both women realised independently of one another, even when adults were crushed by poverty or physically incapacitated, and were thought by many to be beyond the reach of reason, they could still give perfectly reasonable responses, if they were addressed like human beings.

Florence may have found that reasoning with vulnerable people came to her easily after years of being considered unreasonable herself. She could talk to prostitutes dying of cholera, or to British soldiers suffering mortal pain, and she was sure it was equally possible to talk to workhouse patients. As she once expressed it passionately in a letter to her father:

> *That to neglect or ill use the imbecile old women, the dirty child, is the same crime of lèse-majesté against the Almighty that blasphemy of God is.*[1]

For years, she had been concerned about the need for good nurses in workhouse infirmaries. Then, in 1896, she was consulted by Julia Ann Elizabeth Roundell, a writer who asked her to check a speech Roundell had drafted to give to nurses working in workhouse infirmaries. Florence approved the speech, and took the opportunity to share with Roundell some thoughts of her own:

> *There is so much to be done for Workh*[ouse]*: Patients. Nurses always dread the Infirm Wards, where the old Patients have to be 'changed' 5 or 6 times in a night. But a good and clever Nurse will, after nursing them like children, treat them like reasonable beings.* [She gave an example of a nurse chatting to an old woman.] *And the old woman is so delighted. She says 'O you know all about me.'*[2]

Florence must have had similarly reasonable conversations at Scutari. With her, a soldier would feel that he was more than a body wracked with pain. His being could be calmed when she talked to him gently. Accounts of Florence agree on her calm manner and soft voice. One witness reported: 'I have known her [Nightingale] spend hours over men dying of cholera or fever... especially if it was that of a dying man, her slight form would be seen bending over him, administering to his case in every way in her power, and seldom quitting his side till death released him.'[3] She regarded each death as a holy moment when a soul was reunited with its maker. No wonder, then, that the way she nursed sounds so personal and tender. So it's understandable that, back in England, she admitted to having maternal feelings for soldiers, living and dead. It explains why soldiers who survived were so grateful to her, and exchanged stories about her. A few who survived long enough eventually became pall-bearers to her coffin, in 1910.

Before Florence had been a year at Scutari, accounts of her nursing had spread to the poorest classes of English society. Elizabeth, who was familiar with factory workers in Manchester, wrote to Parthenope:

> *Babies ad libitum are being christened Florence here* [in Manchester]*; poor little factory babies, whose grimed stunted parents brighten up at the name, although you'd think their lives*

> *& thoughts were bound up in* [cotton-]*fluffy mills. But it's the old story 'for we have all of us one human heart', & these poor unromantic fellows are made, somehow, of the same stuff as her heroes of the East, who turned their faces to the wall, & cried at her* [Nightingale's] *illness.*[4]

To these factory workers, it didn't matter that Florence was a gentlewoman at a time when class distinctions were rigid and obvious. They recognised, from personal and newspaper accounts that reached them from Scutari, that she genuinely cared about soldiers from their class. She had her own triage system. To the amazement of wounded officers, she did not give them priority treatment, but attended first to those who needed it most.

Even when she was quite young, Florence felt uncomfortable at her gentry status, especially when she was admired for visiting the sick in cottages round Lea Hurst:

> *I had always been in the habit of visiting the poor at home, but it was so unsatisfactory. For me to preach patience to them, when they saw me with what they thought every blessing (ah how little they knew) seemed to me such an impertinence and always checked me... But to visit them in a carriage and give them money is so little like following Christ.*[5]

'She is ambitious – very,' wrote Florence's perceptive sister.[6] And she was. But all her life she eschewed personal grandeur. Her first ambition was to become a trained nurse, to heal those she could, and later to speak truth about hospital and army conditions to power, with enough force to generate some action.

Her life-story shows how difficult it was for her to pursue a goal that her contemporaries thought unreasonable. She had to swim against a powerful mainstream current. Becoming a professional nurse might have looked easy, after she had done it. She showed the way forward for many. But it wasn't easy for her. The pull of this strong mainstream current urges the majority to swim with the tide, to conform, and to doubt whether it is possible to do otherwise. A person who questions whether there is an alternative can feel crazy. Only in retrospect can that sort of question sound reasonable. This was the dilemma that Florence faced. She spent years trying to be an obedient daughter and a kind sister. She was fond of the members of her family as individuals, and depended on them for financial support. They, in turn, depended on her obedience: her mother assured her that, if she became a professional nurse, she would bring dishonour on the whole Nightingale family. Florence was unable to convince her otherwise. It took the British government finally to do that!

But nor could Florence deny her utter certainty that she, personally, had been called on by God to contribute valuable work – work that was destined for herself alone. It would lead her, she was sure, far from her mother's drawing room and elegant conversations. And, although 'I was always expected to be in the drawing room,' she recalled, 'God never left me quite alone.'[7]

As we have seen, her first plan was to get practical nursing experience by visiting Salisbury Infirmary, near the Nightingales' larger house at Embley Park. Her mother was horrified at this idea, and Florence was in despair at such strong opposition. But later she was reasonable enough to see her mother's point. 'I must confess now,' she wrote in 1851, 'that I can understand a mother not liking her daughter to go into an English hospital.'[8] Unfortunately, Mrs Nightingale didn't reciprocate her daughter's understanding. Florence must have undergone many years of being treated as unreasonable. For years, she felt lost. In one of her intimate private notes, dated some time in 1851, she wrote:

> *I what am I* [sic] *that I am not in harmony with all this, that their* [her parents' and sister's] *life is not good enough for me? oh God, what am I? The thoughts & feelings that I have now I can remember since I was 6 years old… the first thought I can remember & the last was nursing work & in the absence of this, education work, but more the education of the bad than of the young.*[9]

Interesting that she felt she could teach 'bad' pupils. Perhaps, as she felt bad herself, she thought she would be able to reach them. In another private note, dated 8 June 1851, she wrote:

> *I have so long struggled to be understood* [by her mother and sister], *been sore, cast down, insupportively fretted by not being understood (at this moment even I feel it when I retrace these conversations in thought) that I must not even try to be understood. I know they can not.*[10]

It took her years to rebuild her inner strength, which seems to have been sapped by her efforts to please her mother and sister. When she visited Kaiserswerth for the second time and with Mrs Nightingale's knowledge, she wrote to her: 'I have not mentioned to anyone where I am... With regard however to your fear of what people will say, the people whose opinions you most care about – it has been their earnest wish for years that I should come here.'[11] So although she had started to fulfil her mission to train as a nurse, she prudently took account of her mother's concern for public opinion.

For Florence, public opinion was secondary. She strove to be guided by what she believed God wanted of her. By the time Elizabeth visited Lea Hurst in 1854, Florence had developed a much stronger conviction that she was on the path God had designed for her. Elizabeth observed:

> *She seems as completely led by God as Joan of Arc... But I never heard of anyone like her – it makes one feel the livingness of God to think how straight He is sending his spirit down into her, as into the prophets & saints of old.*[12]

At first, Florence was alone in her faith that nursing could be transformed from a job undertaken by demoralised, often intoxicated, poor women into a professional career. For all her efforts, she herself had received hardly any training, but she learned how to be organised and competent, as a nurse and as an administrator. In just over a year of working as superintendent of the hospital in Harley Street, she managed to reform the despised job of nursing into a highly skilled vocation. Already, the British government looked to use her nursing and organisational ability. Through her example, nursing quickly became respectable. The Nightingale Fund was established while she was still in Scutari. Only four years after she returned, the Nightingale Home and Training School for Nurses opened in July 1860, as part of St Thomas' Hospital, London. It was the first of its kind in the world.

Before the Crimean War, Florence had a difficult relationship with her mother. From the war onwards, she and her mother wrote regular letters to one another, usually about uncontroversial, practical plans. Florence always signed hers, even when she was in her fifties, 'Your loving child'. After 1870, her mother became demented and eventually blind. Florence spent time looking after her. To her great credit, instead of dismissing her mother as senile, she observed her and managed to find a way to communicate with her. In a 'Most Private' note to her father, she wrote:

> *This sort of conversation only arises when she is lying quite quietly in bed & I am sitting close to her quite quietly. Never when she is walking about the room, or when she makes me walk about the room looking at things. Then, her mind seems utterly to fail her. The most painful confusion of mind arises – in which she often makes the most painful mistakes & remarks... I have observed it now so much as to be quite sure of it.*[13]

'*This*' is not explained, but presumably stands in contrast to the times when Fanny Nightingale's mind failed her. Soon after, in 1874, Florence's father died. Lea Hurst had been entailed to a male heir, but Florence managed to save the house, so that her mother could stay there in comfort. During her mother's helpless years, Parthenope had married and had become absorbed in the Verney family. So Florence, with her quick compassion for those who needed her, left her home in South Street to support her mother at Lea Hurst. It was frustrating for her. She knew she had much work to do.

After the Crimean War, Florence became an activist, if that is the right word to describe a woman who spent decades working from her bedroom. She was haunted and energised by her memories of courageous and uncomplaining grateful soldiers. She felt it was her sacred duty to ensure that in future all soldiers should serve in hygienic conditions, and she was ruthless in demanding that their superiors take genuine responsibility for them. She compared her ideal of a 'moral Army' with the real army and with herself 'struggling daily, hourly, with the selfishness, indifference, wilful resistance' of military chiefs.[14] However, she didn't give up on them. Just as she did with her patients, she appealed to their reason. She was a tireless researcher, and, as we saw in Chapter 8, learned how to show her results visually in statistics that were clear to the eye. Politicians and heads of army staff, however unwilling, had to take account of her. She had enemies, too, who feared her and schemed against her. Victorian society was based on the authority of men. Yet she – a woman – fought for men's respect, and won it.

Florence is one of a few female pioneers who helped to create an alternative way of being a woman in the 19th century. Her friend Sidney Herbert, then secretary at war, recognised her strength of character and predicted what a difference she would make. In a letter he wrote to her, dated 15 October 1854, he said that he hoped she would agree to take a party of nurses to Scutari. She was, he believed, the 'one person in England capable of organising and supervising such a scheme.' He said that, if she accepted:

> *A prejudice will have been broken through and a precedent established which would multiply the good to all times.*[15]

How right he was!

Elizabeth, too, in her letters and publications, appealed to reason. Unlike Florence, she wasn't fighting to reform social injustices, so evident in Manchester. She was sensitive to their complexity. She talked to the very poor, the newly rich, and the landed gentry. Her novels were intended to heighten her readers' awareness of social injustices, taking time to consider them from different viewpoints. Her narrative 'voice' is maternal. It probably isn't the voice that people today want to hear.

Her wonderful *My Diary*, though now published in *Private Voices*, is almost unknown. However, her novels have been dramatised and made into successful films. She originally composed many of her works to be published in serial form in *Household Words, The Cornhill Magazine,* and other journals. So she learned to create plots with chapters that end in suspense. It is tempting to rush through her books or to watch the films only to see how all the romances she set up were resolved. But her novels are much more than their romantic plots. She has insights to communicate on many levels. Through her characters, she shows her understanding of family and societal dilemmas.

From Elizabeth's correspondence, it's clear that she gave out a generous warmth. She attracted people to her. She was maternal, if one can use that word without implying that she was cosy and all-accepting. She studied the people she met, as she had studied her daughters, curious to learn about each. At Lea Hurst, she found plenty to admire in Florence, but still had one criticism. She wrote: 'She is, I think, too much for institutions, sisterhoods and associations.'[16] This was before Florence went to Scutari, so Elizabeth was probably thinking of her hospital work, and her visit to the Sisters of Charity in Paris in 1853, to seek training as a nurse. It was perceptive of Elizabeth to realise that Florence wanted to organise on a large scale. By contrast, Elizabeth's concern was with individuals. When she wrote about a crowd, she nearly always focused on one or two individuals within it.

From *My Diary*, we can see how much Elizabeth learned from her daughters. She could see how different her second daughter was from her first, and yet she loved both of them. Each was special in her own way. From this understanding, she found that she could relate to the wide variety of individuals that she met, exactly as they were. She listened attentively to the way they spoke, and developed an extraordinary ability to create convincing characters in her novels. None is stereotypical. She had an exceptional ear for sound, and gave each an individual voice. Her novels are polyphonic.

Mary Barton is a story set among the rich and poor in Manchester. In one scene, she describes a meeting between 'the masters' of the cotton mills and a delegation of 'the men'. She catches some individual voices of the masters, mostly complacent and scornful of their workmen, though one was more sympathetic. She then introduces the deputation of five workers by their sound: 'Tramp, tramp, came the heavy clogged feet up the stairs.' She adds tiny heart-breaking details that indicate their poverty. After the meeting, one of the workmen admits to the others: 'I'm obligated to pin my waistcoat up, to hide that I've gotten no shirt.'[17]

By the time Elizabeth wrote *Wives and Daughters*, which was to be her last and unfinished novel, she could express the nature of each character in a few words, and trust her readers to understand the logic that continued to guide their ideas and actions. She could convey not just the sound of their individual voices, but their relationship to one another. This is evident in an exchange between Lord and Lady Cumnor, a highly respected earl and his wife:

> *He* [Lord Cumnor] *came up to her and put his hand on her shoulder.*
> *'I'm afraid you're sadly tired, my lady,' he said.*
> *She braced her muscles, and drew herself up, saying coldly, –*
> *'When I am tired, Lord Cumnor, I will tell you so.'*[18]

Elizabeth must have enjoyed writing that! But she goes on to show that Lady Cumnor was expressing a false pride. Lord Cumnor was right. His wife *was* tired. It's a good example of a marriage, showing how Lord Cumnor had a much more casual ability to admit to his own weaknesses than his wife, who disconcerted those around her when she stood on her dignity.

Wives and Daughters is an unusual novel. It contains two

important weddings and two funerals. Readers are told about the preparations for them, but not invited to witness them. Instead, it's the drama of daily life that fills the pages.

With a single word, Elizabeth exposes the style of one of the main characters in *Wives and Daughters*. This is Mrs Kirkpatrick, a widow, who is engaged to marry Mr Gibson. He is the local doctor, himself a widower. Their wedding is soon to take place.

> *Mr Gibson believed that Cynthia Kirkpatrick* [Mrs Kirkpatrick's daughter by her first husband] *was to return to England to be present at her mother's wedding; but Mrs Kirkpatrick had no such intention. She was not what is commonly called a woman of determination; but somehow what she disliked she avoided, and what she liked she tried to do, or to have.*[19]

It is the 'somehow' that warns Elizabeth's readers of the indirect manner in which Mrs Kirkpatrick/Gibson will get her way. Of course, Cynthia did not come to the wedding.

When Elizabeth wrote *My Diary*, her children were young. But by the time the first instalment of *Wives and Daughters* was published, it was August 1864. Marianne was now a woman of nearly 30. Elizabeth had had plenty of time to reflect on her mothering and to ask herself how far the influence of a mother's early decisions can affect the development of a child into adulthood. She doesn't imply that a mother's influence would determine the fate of her child. Rather she was curious to find out whether she could see a connection. As she unwinds the various threads of *Wives and Daughters*, she is able to show what she has learned.

Mr Gibson, the widowed doctor, has one child, his daughter, Molly. She is 17 when his new wife and, a bit later, her daughter Cynthia, come to live with them. Readers already know that Molly's mother fell ill and died when Molly was less than four years old. Now Molly's father has married Cynthia's mother, formerly Mrs Kirkpatrick. Their daughters are about the same age. They get to know one another and form a strong friendship. But Cynthia is quick to notice a difference between Molly and herself. She confesses: '"I wish I could love people as you do, Molly... A good number of people love me, I believe, or at least they think they do; but I never seem to care much for any one."'

Looking back on her childhood, Cynthia then reflects:

> *I was a trouble, I daresay. So I was sent to school at four years old; first one school, and then another; and in the holidays, mamma went to stay at grand houses, and I was generally left with the schoolmistresses... Somehow I cannot forgive her* [Cynthia's mother] *for her neglect of me as a child, when I would have clung to her. Besides, I hardly ever heard from her when I was at school.*[20]

Elizabeth had already warned her readers that 'somehow what she [Mrs Kirkpatrick] disliked she avoided'. So now readers can see this avoidance in action. 'I was a trouble,' ventures Cynthia. But all children are 'a trouble' – or, rather, require a good deal of care. When Mrs Kirkpatrick would not let Cynthia cling to her, she was depriving her young daughter of a basic mammalian need. It is understandable, then, that Cynthia had grown up, unable to forgive her mother for her neglect, still yearning to be loved (acting seductively towards men to get a substitute for that need), but found that she could not love in return. Cynthia's situation makes a significant contrast to Molly's. Molly's mother had died when she was young, but hadn't neglected her. Molly cherished the few memories she had of her mother. So, unlike Cynthia, she found it easy to love.

Many mothers in fiction are either absent (as Florence Nightingale pointed out, see page 81), or selfish and self-centred. In *Wives and Daughters,* Lady Cumnor and Mrs Gibson are both mothers who are unquestionably self-centred. Yet there are scenes in which Elizabeth reveals their more generous sides. In the same realistic way, she depicts an essentially good mother, Mrs Hamley, who loves her children yet is far from ideal. It is worth taking a close look at Mrs Hamley. Both she and Mrs Gibson profess to love and care for Molly. Elizabeth does not contrast them herself, but leaves her readers to draw their own conclusions.

Elizabeth introduces Mrs Hamley's husband first, the robust Tory, Squire Roger Hamley, of the ancient family at Hamley Hall. Mrs Hamley, explains Elizabeth, is: 'a delicate London lady; it was one of those perplexing marriages of which one cannot understand the reasons.'[21] Squire Hamley is a proud man who feels educationally inferior to his wife and her friends. Eventually 'she gave up her visits to London; she gave up her social pleasure in the company of her fellows in education and position.' After that, though never becoming exactly ill, she is never quite well. She has two sons, and a daughter who died young. Readers aren't told whether it might have been childbirth, in addition to the sacrifice of her London life, that has weakened her. She is, after all, introduced as 'delicate'.

As the novel unfolds, Mrs Hamley grows weaker and dies, as do so many gentle mothers in Elizabeth's work. It would be easy to write her off as a mother who died early because she made too great a sacrifice of her own needs for the sake of her family. Jenny Uglow, one of Elizabeth's biographers, describes Mrs Hamley as a woman who 'suppresses her own interests', and who, in life, endures 'a living death'.[22]

Mrs Hamley is a contrast to Elizabeth herself. Elizabeth recovered from several serious illnesses, and suffered acutely from neuralgia for many years.[23] But she had irrepressible resources of energy which she used for writing, as well as for meeting her friends, and travelling to London and abroad, often with one of her daughters.

The fictional Mrs Hamley also has energy, but of a different kind. After Mrs Hamley's death, Elizabeth, as her author, reveals a deeper understanding of the mother she has created.

> *Quiet and passive as Mrs Hamley had always been in appearance, she was the ruling spirit of the house as long as she lived. The*

> *directions to the servants, down to the most minute particulars, came from her sitting-room, or from the sofa on which she lay. Her children always knew where to find her; and to find her was to find love and sympathy. Her husband, who was often restless and angry from one cause or another, always came to her to be smoothed down and put right... But the keystone of the family arch was gone, and the stones of which it was composed began to fall apart.*[24]

'The keystone of the family arch' is a brilliant and original metaphor to describe a mother. It gives her a strong position, requiring a special energy that may not be visible, but can be felt by those around her. She could have exploited her position to control the family. But Elizabeth assures her readers that Mrs Hamley's family received not control, but her love. So was this a form of self-sacrifice?

Mrs Hamley's 'fellows in education and position' in London must have provided some fine intellectual stimulation. But, in time, this can feel insufficient. In marrying Squire Hamley, a marriage that was considered 'perplexing', Mrs Hamley received some advantages that could not be matched by a London intellectual life. She gained a secure and peaceful home, a husband who cherished her, and the love of her sons.

She certainly gave up her social life. But she kept alive her interests. Elizabeth explains that Mrs Hamley always had, on a table beside her, the newest books of poetry and fiction, together with loose sheets of blank paper. She would lie on a sofa, in a room looking out onto flower gardens, a lily pond and the Hamley woods. She would read, and write poetry. She took care of her health too. Every three hours, her maid would bring her a draught of medicine, a glass of water, and, adds Elizabeth who loves detail, a biscuit. It sounds a civilised life that Mrs Hamley has chosen.

While their sons are away, studying at Cambridge, Molly comes to stay with the Hamleys. Readers then get a chance to see the 'keystone' energy for themselves. Molly enjoys all the hospitality and tender friendship that Mrs Hamley gives her, and wants to stay with her as often as she can. However, one day Mrs Hamley receives distressing news of her older son, Osborne. Molly is able to give her comfort, and Mrs Hamley exclaims: 'You're a real blessing to mothers, child! You give one such pleasant sympathy, both in one's gladness and in one's sorrow.'[25] On another occasion, Mrs Hamley explains the reasons for her distress, again about Osborne, but also looks into Molly's eyes to catch her 'sympathy from their expression quicker than she could from her words.'[26] When the younger son, Roger, returns home because Mrs Hamley is ill, he mentions the family conflict about Osborne in talking to Molly: 'My mother would have brought us all right, if she'd been what she once was.'[27] So Mrs Hamley definitely was the 'keystone' figure for her family and for Molly. But she received as much as she gave. She gave them a strong form of love, and received love and comfort from them when she needed it.

The Hamleys' two sons are 23 and 21 at the start of the novel. Both parents admire Osborne, the older son, more than Roger, his brother. Osborne wins prizes at school and is expected to do brilliantly at Cambridge. His mother especially prefers him, and Elizabeth makes it clear that Mrs Hamley's excessive devotion to Osborne is harmful to him. Even so, the two boys receive plentiful parental affection, and are fond of one another. As young men, neither has any difficulty falling in love. Osborne loves and secretly marries the appropriately named Aimée (loved). As she was French (an unpopular nationality in England since the Napoleonic Wars), a Roman Catholic, and a mere nursemaid, Osborne does not dare confess his marriage to his father. Roger, the younger son, first falls for the seductive Cynthia but eventually finds that Molly is the one he truly loves. Readers have long been aware that Molly silently loves Roger. It is unfortunate that Elizabeth died before completing the novel. She was an expert at suspense, so there were some misunderstandings between Molly and Roger that she would have planned to resolve. But since she had already written 60 chapters, the novel must have been almost finished, and she told her editor that she meant them to marry.

In *Wives and Daughters*, Elizabeth shows that those who were loved by their parents as young children find it easy to fall in love as young adults. Through Cynthia, she shows how it feels to be seductive but detached. Mr Gibson, as the stepfather responsible for her, points out how much unhappiness her seductive behaviour has caused the men who fall in love with her. Cynthia tells him bitterly that she knows her faults. She continues:

> *Oh, sir, I think if I had been differently brought up I should not have had the same sore angry heart that I have. Now! No don't! I don't want reasoning comfort. I can't stand it. I should always have wanted admiration and worship and men's good opinion.*[28]

This idea – that neglect of a small girl could adversely affect her ability to love when she was older – was Elizabeth's. It derived from her own observations. Elizabeth also shows that Cynthia's desire for 'admiration and worship' was no substitute for mutual love. In most of Elizabeth's novels, there are long-married couples who continue to love one another, and benefit from their shared companionship and mutual support as they age.

Her novels have many themes running through them. One of these is of a wrongdoing, acknowledgement, and reconciliation. Even a cruel person, thought Elizabeth, could redeem themselves if they repented of their wrongdoings. 'The most depraved,' she wrote, 'have also their Seed of the Holiness that shall one day overcome their evil.'[29] It was only a tiny seed, as yet undeveloped, as she saw it. But she had faith that the seed held unrealised potential for the highest good.

In nearly all her novels, there is a powerful, self-righteous, judgemental man. As the plot unfolds, this man discovers that he has been too harsh towards a weaker character, usually his son. He breaks down in tears of remorse, acknowledges his love for his son, and concedes that his judgements have been too strict. He begs forgiveness and to be reconciled, if this is possible. The fiery Squire

Hamley is one such character.

All these scenes of paternal remorse are intimate and moving. No longer powerful and judgemental, the man is re-humanised and restored to being a person who can love. It's interesting that these scenes recur in Elizabeth's work. (*Wives and Daughters* also contains a contrasting very tender scene in which Roger Hamley insists on smoking a friendly pipe together with his irascible father, the Squire, also called Roger.)[30]

How far did Elizabeth believe that those two-person reconciliation moments, between a powerful father and his problematic son, could be extended to reconcile conflicts on a much larger scale? Her earlier novels describe calculating cotton-mill owners and their 'clemming' (starving) workers. She was aware of the stark social injustices of her time, of class snobbery, and of the humiliation of the poor. But in her novels, the landed gentry and the self-made mill owners are not inherently heartless, nor are the poor shown as entirely helpless.

A dramatic example of a confrontation between rich and poor occurs in *North and South*. It was written just before Elizabeth came to Lea Hurst. For some time, the workers at the fictional Thornton's cotton mill have been threatening to go on strike. The mill owner, John Thornton, decides to protect his interests by importing some Irish workers to take the strikers' place. This inflames his workmen, and they crowd towards Thornton's home. Elizabeth doesn't mention that they have a leader or a particular plan. It's not clear what the men will do when they get there. Thornton sends out for help from the army, and believes that troops will soon arrive to support him.

By chance, Margaret Hale (the novel's main protagonist) is present at his home. Unusually for a woman of her class, she is not afraid, nor does she support the use of violence to quell the strikers. 'Can you do nothing,' she challenges Thornton, 'to soothe these poor creatures [the mill workers]? It is awful to see them.' Thornton tells her: 'The soldiers will be here directly, and that will bring them to reason.' 'To reason!' exclaims Margaret.

'What kind of reason?' Thornton replies: 'The only reason that does with men that make themselves into wild beasts. By heaven! They've turned to the mill-door!' At this point, Margaret appeals to him:

> *Mr Thornton, go down this instant, if you are not a coward. Go down and face them like a man. Save these poor strangers* [the imported Irish workers] *whom you have decoyed here. Speak to your workmen as if they were human beings. Speak to them kindly. Don't let the soldiers come in and cut down poor creatures who are driven mad.*[31]

These words come from the mouth of 19-year-old Margaret. But she is surely speaking in the humane, maternal voice of Elizabeth herself. She had studied the faces of Manchester mill-hands. She was sure that the fictional workers at Thornton's mill were not really like wild beasts but basically reasonable individuals who were 'driven mad' with fear that their families would starve. And surely 'Speak to them kindly' is the *cri de cœur* of mothers everywhere who have borne children, nurtured them night and day, year after year, hoped for them, feared for them, and desired them to live, to have enough food for their families, and to be safe from the threat of armed soldiers. As Elizabeth wrote to Parthenope: 'for we have all of us one human heart', which is a line from Wordsworth's poem, 'The Old Cumberland Beggar'.[32]

At this stage in *North and South*, trust between master and men has broken down. Both sides are angry and the men are frightened. It might not be the best moment for Thornton to 'speak to them kindly'. But then – who knows?

'Kind' is a useful word. It derives from 'kin' and 'kindred', meaning family or race, so originally 'kind' was used to refer to the feelings that relatives were expected to have for one another. In a wider context, that of the whole human race, it links to Margaret's words: '"Speak to your workmen as if they were human beings."' Florence had a similar idea when she wrote that nurses caring for patients in a workhouse infirmary could 'treat them like reasonable beings'.

However, speaking kindly, humanely and reasonably is not enough. The speaker has to support his words with the ability to listen. Elizabeth was a superb listener, very patient, able to register tones and nuances. Most speakers would need training to be able to listen as openly to two opposing sides as she did. When crowds of cotton-workers surround a mill-owner's home because they face starvation, and when their employer believes they have made themselves into wild beasts, the likelihood is that neither side will give the other a chance. The most common outcome is for the members of each side to raise their voices, accuse the other, and hasten to defend themselves. Neither can relax enough to listen calmly to the 'opposing' side.

Later in *North and South*, Mr Thornton, the proud self-made mill owner, is approached for work by the equally proud workman and union leader, Nicholas Higgins. They don't speak to one another with any kindness whatsoever. They annoy one another greatly, but then, suddenly, they acknowledge this with honesty and humour, and shake hands. After that, Thornton gives Higgins a job. Elizabeth could see how a conflict might be resolved on a personal level. But she must have wondered whether there could be human justice on a larger scale.

Elizabeth and Florence were both, in their different ways, maternal. Both had faith in the ultimate good of humanity. But neither overlooked how selfish people can be. Both believed in appealing to reason as a way of dealing with conflict, with prejudice and the breakdown of trust. Their main difference was one of style.

Florence was not impressed by what she had seen of individual mothers with their children. But, as we saw, she herself cherished deep maternal feelings for groups of people, especially for the soldiers she had nursed at Scutari. Paintings of the war show mature men, but in reality some were only boys in their early teens who had lied about their age so as not to miss the 'glory of war'. Florence cared passionately, not for a few individual soldiers, but for all those she had known. She kept her resolution to fight for better conditions on their behalf. She could be forthright and unyielding, and usually got her way. Yet, 40 years after the end of the war, when she was 76, the memories of those brave soldiers and the unnecessary deprivations they suffered still rankled. Her anger comes through in a note she wrote in about 1896:

> *The troops were living on salt meat, when the finest cattle in the world were swarming on the shores of the Black Sea... Raw coffee was sent out from England, when every man, woman and child in Constantinople had his, her or its cup of coffee every morning. And the* [soldiers] *had* [hard] *biscuits when they might have had any quantity of bread. The troops had only salt meat, biscuit and grog.*[33]

Elizabeth's style was different. She loved peace, and knew that it was necessary to work for it. Her novels are filled with conflicts based on misunderstanding. Once a misunderstanding has arisen, all subsequent situations seem to confirm it, and it takes a good deal of thought and patience to re-establish the truth. Elizabeth believed in the complexity of open discussion rather than the simplicity of a single-minded attack, which Florence favoured. But their ideas were similar. In *Mary Barton*, Elizabeth wrote:

> *No one thought of treating the workmen as brethren and friends, and openly, clearly, as appealing to reasonable men, stating the exact and full circumstances, which led the masters to think that it was the wise policy of the time to make sacrifices themselves; and to hope for them from the operatives.*[34]

'No one' meant the masters, the mill owners. Elizabeth thought that if they could treat their workmen as brothers and friends, and if they would explain the reasons for their policies, then they could hope that their workmen would be equally reasonable and understand. She didn't claim to have all the answers. But she believed that a human conversation would be a good start. After all, masters and men alike needed the cotton mills to survive.

So what happened to the 'grand quarrel'? The issue of whether there should be crèches for the rich as well as for the poor was important to both Elizabeth and Florence. They don't appear to have resolved this difference. But Elizabeth's admiration for Florence never abated, while Florence changed her mind over the escapist nature of novels, and also seems to have abandoned her idea about crèches. So, after the Crimean War, the two exchanged books they had written, and cooperated over special projects together. It's a great pity that they didn't revisit their conflict.

The two sides of the 'grand quarrel' are relevant today. The different perspectives that Elizabeth and Florence brought to it can help us to clarify what is at stake. But there are underlying values that both shared. Both had faith in our common humanity, and both believed in every person's ability to respond to kindness and reason. The two sides to their quarrel, and their underlying shared values, take us to Chapter 10.

II

Mothers Today

Chapter 10

Where have all the mothers gone?

It was sad to hear a mother admit recently: 'You feel you are second class as a mother.'

Though it's not surprising. The revolutionary vision of Florence Nightingale, that women were capable of (or were designed by God for) much more than keeping home and caring for their children, has been realised. Other women were as determined about this as she was. Increasingly, around the world, women have been educated, trained and employed. They now own their earnings, and open bank accounts. No longer need they depend financially on their fathers or husbands. This has become a normal part of everyday life. Women have gained immeasurably.

The pendulum has swung in Western countries since the time of the 'grand quarrel'. Unfortunately, instead of coming to rest in the middle, it has swung way out to the other side. Instead of women now having a genuine choice as to whether to become fulltime mothers, to work fulltime outside their homes, or to mix the two, they now find it relatively straightforward to do fulltime paid work, but much harder to afford fulltime motherhood while their children are young. The reality is that the 'Nightingales' are now in a much stronger position than the 'Gaskells'.

But are all women alike? Nightingale and the feminists who followed believed that every woman should be freed from the limitations of home. However, not every mother feels limited in her home. Some find a different kind of freedom and independence *within* it. Home doesn't have to feel like a trap. It can be a sanctuary, separate from the world of commerce. A mother can enjoy the freedom in the privacy of home to develop her own values and to bring up her family as she sees best.

Within their homes, mothers can prepare their children for the complexities of modern social life. Above all, children need to know the joy of being loved and having their love accepted. The relationships they form with their mothers are intimate. Without these relationships – and young children need a lot of love – life can easily feel pointless.

Many children today learn how to survive in groups, sometimes from babyhood. Group skills differ from maternal one-to-one intimacy. Nightingale's brainwave of having crèches for the rich as well as for the poor – which must have sounded crazy when she voiced it to Gaskell – has become reality. The government pays for a limited amount of childcare, while private crèches and nurseries are available for anyone who can pay for them. Mothers are encouraged to return promptly to their employed work and to use a relative, nursery or crèche for daily childcare. However, this gives them less time to continue the warm, intimate connection many have formed with their children. When these mothers return to paid work, they describe constant pangs of guilt.

Our society is organised for mothers to bear children, but not to look after them. The outcome has been not to liberate mothers from home, but to increase the economic output of each nation. What looked like more freedom for mothers has slowly played into the interests of the market economies of different countries.

This can be confusing for a young woman. Her education has prepared her to earn her living, to be ambitious at work, but not to become a mother. Many new mothers look back at their education, and realise how little all-round preparation they were given. For example:

> *It's counter-cultural. I was raised to think about career only. I heard lots about women 'smashing the glass ceiling'. Nowhere was raising a family mentioned.*

> *I've been casting my mind back to my schooldays and in sex-ed the assumption was that children are an obstacle to the noble*

process of self-actualisation.[1]

I believe that at this moment in time Western women are the least prepared we have ever been for maternity leave and becoming mothers. We have been raised to shoot for the moon career-wise.[2]

Many teachers have promoted the mainstream feminist perspective, especially the idea that spending time mothering a child would be a waste of a valuable education. From this position, it would be a retrograde step for a schoolgirl to ignore all the liberty and freedom that was fought for on her behalf. Doesn't she betray her feminism if she plans to have a family? Alex Jones, a female journalist, described this predicament:

Throughout school, throughout your teenage years, throughout your twenties, the main thing is: 'don't get pregnant because that will mess up your career'... Nobody at any point said, 'but you might want to think about it [getting pregnant] *if you want a family because, actually, it is as important as a career'. I thought it was a bit unfeminist in a way even to say, 'I'm worried about my fertility' because you're so busy carving out your career.*[3]

A girl may leave school or college, competent at reading, mathematics, and other essentials to apply for a job or start a career. It may look like an exciting and liberating world that she is entering, with plenty of opportunities. To some extent, it is. Employers are usually glad to use her skills in exchange for regular payments, and often for the security of a retirement pension. And she can feel she is learning more useful skills and extending her abilities. She may be satisfied with this. But the difficulty is that she has entered a commercial world with its own values and demands. It is not nearly as generous to her as it might first appear.

Modern society is based on economic viability, and it's convenient for many companies to retain their trained and valuable female members of staff. A new mother is often told that she is needed back in the workforce soon after her baby is born. She may well need the money. She may also be trained, experienced and take pleasure in doing her job. She may find her paid work much easier than caring for her newborn. Her employers and colleagues want to retain her, and claim that they can't do without her. Their generous comments can be very persuasive. Yet, however excellent she was at her job, she can usually be replaced, even if her substitute is not quite so capable. It may be difficult for her to realise that, as a mother, her unique voice, her smell, her touch, her rhythm – these are special for her baby.

One experienced mother wrote:

> *Mums aren't really told how important they are to their children and they go blindly with tired eyes back to the life they had before.*

Most new mothers take maternity leave. But this term suggests that a woman is getting a special concession from her employer, like her 'annual leave' which is holiday. It can tie her to her employers. Once she has a baby, she may depend on them financially, as much as her unliberated great-grandmother depended on *her* father and husband.

This dilemma is very rarely discussed. The birth-rate is declining worldwide. Societies are concerned to reproduce themselves. So women are encouraged to *have* children but not to continue bringing them up. Not all women want to have children. Those who have families may not want to spend time bringing them up, but blend their jobs or careers with childcare.

The tragedy is that there *are* mothers who want to devote more time to their children, at least for the early years. Many return to their employment because that's what is expected of them. They've chosen nurseries, they are under contract to return, and their decisions now seem inevitable. And yet many are not nearly as compliant as they might appear. 'Up to 78% of parents with children under five,' concludes the organisation Mothers At Home Matter, 'would like to spend more time with their children, but feel they cannot afford to. Less than one in four mothers can afford to be at home to care for their own young children.' 'It's a luxury I can't afford,' mothers say. But should this important decision be made for financial reasons alone?

These mothers lose out, their children lose out, and our society then lacks the benefit, later on, of secure adults whose mothers enjoyed caring for them as children. Unfortunately, too many children witness how concerned their parents are with their paid work. This, in turn, may result in their growing into adulthood feeling of little worth unless they, too, are earning money. A person's sense of having *intrinsic* value usually develops from humane early mothering. There are other ways, but there isn't a better way.

The media publish very negative impressions of motherhood. If I were a schoolgirl, trying to imagine my future, these reports would definitely put me off.

> *A lot of parenting is also basically grunt work that is both mind-numbingly boring and repetitive, from the feeding to the endless laundry, to the homework chivvying...But as well as this you have to be able to meet all of your child's emotional needs, to acknowledge that everything is all your fault, but also to be able to fix it.*[4]

> *It's true that parents sacrifice sleep, sanity and the distant memory of having once had plans of their own in return for stinking nappies, a household of plastic tat, and the chance to provide a free taxi service for grunting ingrates.*[5]

Some women identify with the role they have in their paid employment. Living with their newborns doesn't suit them at all. Paid work gives them a sense of their own value, which they don't get from being mothers. For example:

> *Now I am a mother with a delicious peach of a five-week-old daughter. She is addictively cute to me, gorgeous and lovable. But*

do I feel that 'bringing her to earth' was 'empowering'? Far from it. Work is what makes me feel empowered and that is why I am continuing to do it even as my baby sleeps on my chest in a sling.[6]

We (stay-at-home mums) are just different varieties of parasite... I basically don't believe that anyone will want to hire me. Some days, I doubt that I have any marketable skills whatsoever.[7]

A common aggressive question is: 'Why do women have children if they don't want to look after them?' It's not easy to predict how a woman will feel after her baby is born. It may be only after giving birth that a new mother discovers her real feelings. Each of us has a particular life-history, and this affects us. As one mother put it: 'Everyone [i.e. every mother] arrives in a different way.' She was close to tears as she remembered:

In the beginning I thought my baby was a huge mistake. I just wished someone would come and take her away.

Teachers, who have done such excellent work in persuading girls that they could learn maths and science as intelligently as their brothers, seem to have had a more collective powerful influence on young girls than each individual teacher might realise. A career is presented as worthy of a woman's abilities, while becoming a mother is often regarded as demeaning. Lucy Jones, in her book *Matrescence*, expresses succinctly what many women feel:

Until matrescence, I had sought to live a life like my father's. Now, I found myself living my mother's life. I had switched from protagonist to stagehand.[8]

A stagehand simply moves the props that the main actors will need. Jones felt she had become a background member of the working team, no longer one of the leading characters. That was her expectation *before* her experience of having three children. Did she change her mind *after* having them? In her Epilogue, six years later, she used the same image of a theatre to sum up her position. She says that, since publishing *Matrescence*, many women have contacted her to say that she has articulated how they feel too. So her view is likely to be a common one:

> *My children are the main actors, and I am the audience. I will always be in thrall to them, but they won't always be in thrall to me.*[9]

Perhaps, as I am a grandmother, I can offer a more balanced perspective. In my experience, and from what many mothers tell me, I have found that they and their children develop reciprocal relationships. Children study their mothers in minute detail. They are then the 'audience', to keep to Jones's image, watching their mothers in action. Children learn what to expect of life from their mothers. Jones expresses her love when she says that she will always be in thrall to her children. But, if the relationship develops well, children love their mothers with generous warmth. A mother's love seems to sustain her child for a lifetime, while she, perhaps aware of her many faults, is grateful for signs that her child continues to love her too.

At the moment, negative views of motherhood predominate. Mothers who have enjoyed the experience are reluctant to say so, perhaps out of fear of attracting ridicule or accusations of being smug and boastful. One mother reflected this by writing what she herself thought in brackets.

> *We've become too 'civilised' or 'clean cut' or important to care for our own kids. They are too dirty, too difficult to deal with. It's frightening filling the hours with them. Why would intelligent women do it? It's seen as a retrograde step or beneath us somehow. (It's not beneath me.)*

Why *would* an intelligent woman care for her own children? If we look closely, we shall see that our society doesn't have a problem with *starting* to be a mother. Women are encouraged to give birth, and to 'settle' their babies for their early months. Newborns often have long stretches of sleep during their first weeks, but once they are awake they can't be left alone. That's a lot for a mother to do, during her maternity leave.

But what happens *after* that? Hasn't she done the main part of her job? The rest is daily maintenance and repetition, surely. Doesn't it make sense for an intelligent mother to return to her paid work?

One of the first questions that new mothers ask one another is: 'When are you going back to work?' The expectation is that each will soon return. It can feel comforting. Life with a newborn may feel very odd compared to the more structured work these women are used to. Western society isn't mother-friendly, and all mothers face some difficulties. So when mothers meet, they are often curious about how each is managing. They may sit round a cafe table, or stand in the street. If you or I walk past, we might hear bursts of laughter as they turn their unfortunate mishaps of mothering into hilarious stories, and then there's a silence when we suddenly see that one of them is crying. The others comfort her. It's obvious that they value one another's support.

They soon discover that they have certain anxieties in common. Solveig Brown, an American researcher, interviewed 40 mothers. She describes what she learned:

> *When I asked women what is the hardest thing about being a mother, many mothers spoke of feeling guilty because they frequently wonder if they are saying or doing the right thing, and nearly every mother reported feeling under pressure or stressed.*[10]

It takes time for a mother to discover that there is rarely one 'right thing' that she should be doing. But if her maternity leave is short, she may never learn this. When mothers agree to a fixed-length maternity leave, which may be unavoidable, it may also set up an emotional barrier. Knowing that she will have to return to paid work may make it harder for a mother to allow herself to fall in love with her child. The awareness that she will soon give her child to professional day care can inhibit her.

For some mothers, an early return to work is what they had always intended. But for many, it's a dilemma. They describe the wrench they feel when it's time to leave their children. Before giving birth, a mother might have thought that she had signed up to a generous amount of maternity leave. Now, some months later, she can see how much her child still needs her. How will he manage without her understanding? Hardly anyone but herself will recognise what he is trying to say. (I'm using the male pronoun for a child to avoid confusion with the mother.)

When the time comes to leave her child at nursery, the mother will often report that he clung to her and cried at having to let her go. That's exactly the development that an earlier return to work is designed to avoid. Mothers and children aren't expected to become too attached. Children are praised as 'good' when they can be taken from one setting to another, without tears and clinging. Once the mother has detached herself and left for paid work, she will usually be assured by a message from the nursery staff that her child has settled down well, and is playing happily. Whereas she, while trying to focus on her work, may worry about her child all day. Both she and her child may be putting brave faces on a situation that they feel powerless to change.

It takes considerable courage for a mother to step 'out of line' and decide to care for her child beyond her maternity leave. Some use their savings. Some are self-employed, which makes the decision easier. But what do mothers experience when they cross the invisible barrier and enter into *dis*couraged territory?

It's easy to be daunted. Mothers sense the social stigma if they resign from their jobs to spend more time with their children. They fear that they will be judged negatively, and even worry that they will be pathologised for appearing to lose their separate identities and becoming 'slaves' to their children. As one mother wrote:

> *The culture remains that you should juggle work and kids (somehow); for a career woman to 'give up' work when you have children, as I did, is seen as rather embarrassing, if not an outright failure.*

We have to listen to what mothers say to appreciate just how difficult it is to step away from the economic pressures of our society. The first steps are especially hard, not only financially but emotionally too. A new mother may feel crazy to find that she is no longer respected as someone contributing to the national economy. Most mothers go through a period of disorientation which can feel intolerable. That disorientation may be misread as post-natal depression, but it seems to be a more subtle process than that. As one mother put it:

> *I feel I'm in a different reality to other people that they can't see. It feels lonely. I don't have the words for it. It's* visceral, *that's the nature of motherhood.*

Visceral is a physical word. One dictionary defines it as: 'felt, or as if, in the internal organs of the body.' The mother must have felt she was experiencing a deep inner change.

Many mothers say, as she did, that it's hard to find the words to explain this. They weren't expecting to love their babies so profoundly, nor to want more time to care for them. 'But I've been right through birth,' mothers may think. 'Why did no one warn me about after?' They say it's as though they have crossed over from a familiar landscape for which they had been prepared – of having a job and earning a living – to an unknown one of being unprepared and responsible for developing children. Many protest that they feel 'untethered', or that they are 'in a foreign country', or even 'in another dimension'. They feel alone, visible to other people and yet not understood by them.

When does this process start? Some mothers experience the change during pregnancy. They realise that they have already started to communicate with their unborn babies. Tara Ulbrich provides a vivid example:

> *Women have been told to fear losing themselves in motherhood but what if the complete opposite is true? It is possible to find oneself?... When my son was born I realised that though our one body was now two, we were intertwined in a physical connection that was not the same as his connection to his father. My son was breastfed but it was more than this. My body felt a biochemistry beyond that precious self-regulating, milky nurturing. I felt responsible for using this maternal intensity to make something bigger than the two of us and its source lay in this profound womb-knowing of one another.*[11]

Ulbrich struggled to put into words the excitement of her discovery. Her neologism, 'this profound *womb-knowing* of one another' describes her sense of retaining her own identity while sharing a strong pre-natal communication with her son. After all, 'mother' is a *relational* word. It expresses a connection between at least two separate individuals. Even before the birth, when her baby turns over in the amniotic fluid, a mother can feel a rippling inside her. These movements aren't visible, so someone in conversation with her might have no idea that there is a third party 'present'. As Ulbrich says, the mother already has a 'physical connection' with her child. But it might sound strange to anyone who hasn't experienced it.

This is an example of communication that only a biological mother could have. But adoptive mothers have their own ways of creating relationships. One adoptive mother gave this account:

> *I adopted my son when he was eleven months. But he regressed. He needed all that early mothering that he had missed. He couldn't progress without it. When I gave him what he needed, he could move on.*

It was brilliant of her to notice that her son was regressing. Also, perhaps she needed to *give* the early mothering as much as he needed to receive it. Both of them had missed it. She probably held him, skin-to-skin, and enabled the two of them to experience the warm pre-verbal contact that is so important. And that may have enabled them both to move forwards.

Taking on any new job means there is much to learn. Becoming a mother may not seem like starting a new job – haven't most mothers left their jobs for maternity *leave*? – but that's what it is. What a new mother needs is not too much advice or manuals of instructions, but the confidence of people around her that she will learn to manage in her own way. The beginning often feels like a plunge into chaos, but it gets easier in stages.

The lost, disorientated feeling is temporary. Humans are brilliant at recognising patterns even in a chaos of behaviour. Mothers can do this and so, apparently, can their babies. Gradually mothers and babies become more familiar with one another. After several months, they seem to come through the unpredictable chaos, and reach a stage of knowing approximately what to expect.

After years of experience, a woman can feel more confident. But it's hard for her to pass on any wisdom that helped her at the start. I've heard many mothers say that they followed their own instincts. But this doesn't work for every mother.

> First mother: *I didn't know what to do when I had my first child. People were always telling me: 'Just follow your instincts.' But I didn't have any instincts. I was bewildered.*
>
> Second mother: *I'm so glad you said that about not having instincts. You look like the sort of mother who would have them. I didn't have any instincts either.*

This is a good example of the way one mother can take comfort from another. Because – how easy is it to move from a job or fast-moving career environment to a much slower mothering one with such minimal preparation? A mother can't make this transition overnight. It takes time. And the change isn't automatic. The next two mothers both use the words 'allow myself', showing that they each made an active decision about whether to adjust to motherhood.

> *Through having my children, I've allowed myself to change and be this new identity. A life-altering event... why not let yourself be altered?*

> *I am realising that somehow in our post-feminist culture, women are often afraid of motherhood and of the changes that it will bring. I realise that I have embraced those changes, not because I am especially strong or follow some particular parent-orientated philosophy, but because I am simply looking out for my infant. Allowing myself to fall in love with my firstborn helped me to see how much babies need their mothers.*[12]

The first mother could afford to stay at home while her children were young. The second was a self-employed stand-up comedian who took her young children on stage with her at evening shows. They are good examples of the many ways mothers can adapt their lives to include their children.

There is no other relationship like it. The mother needs patience to notice what her child needs. She quickly discovers how sensitive he is to noises and smells that she may take for granted. At first, he may not even know that the people around him are talking to one another. Usually, it's his mother who introduces him to the possibility of communication. This starts long before he can speak. He may not realise that his gestures can be understood. Once his mother starts to respond to him, he receives an early sense of the to-and-fro of communication. Like Gaskell, a new mother may be surprised to discover that her baby is not making random movements, but rather indicating his feelings: that he is bored, or hungry, or excited, or overtired, or something else. One mother announced:

> *She's six months. I sometimes get a little hunch of what she wants.*

Once the mother has 'a little hunch' she can start to test whether she is right. This wonderful moment marks the birth of two-way communication. It's this first step that is especially hard for mothers to learn. Yet the mother has started her child on the long road towards the adult world of complex conversations. Our civilisation would be in chaos without enough mothers doing this work.

Outsiders are unlikely to realise that so much genuine work is going on. Mothers can feel misunderstood and unappreciated. One mother of older children saw, in retrospect, that having children suddenly brought her into conflict with the values of her society.

> *You feel you are second class as a mother. I'm home-schooling, but I feel guilty all the time for not working. And yet there are these amazing beings that come out of your vagina. It makes you kind of flip all your beliefs.*

What beliefs had this mother flipped? Although she was home-schooling, she still felt 'second class' in response to the way other people saw her. Her children were supposed to be at school, and she in paid work. And yet she is not the only mother to find her beliefs 'flip' once she sees her baby. She may have been warned that she would soon get bored as a mother and long to return to her paid work. But when she sees that an 'amazing being' has emerged from her body, she may feel a strong loving curiosity about her child. Suddenly, caring for this person doesn't seem boring at all.

A new kind of mother is emerging. She is not the frustrated kind that Nightingale saw, nor even like most mothers of the 20th century. She is conscious of her worth as a mother. It's interesting that these mothers, who eventually sound sure of themselves, seem to be the very same ones that struggled with feeling lost in the early months. They are similar to Gaskell, who wrote that she was 'so unknowing'. Again, like Gaskell, they seem to have found their own answers. Without coordinating with one another, they seem to have come to similar conclusions. They have resisted the idea that they are supposed to 'manage' their children. They aren't struggling to placate, pacify or silence them. Instead, they see even babies as fellow persons. Some of these mothers are fulltime, while others are employed and have to make the most of their spare time with their children. But all of them can see how essential their maternal work really is.

The common descriptive word 'childcare' seems to suggest the practical and visible tasks that the mother is doing, rather than all the thinking she has done before her actions. Questions that require decisions arise constantly. It's exhausting for a mother to see how many options she has, to weigh them up and to choose one. Some decisions are trivial, but others have long-term consequences. One tired mother explained:

> *People don't realise how much mothers are thinking. The amount of thought I put into what I'm doing amazes me. Every single one of those endless micro-decisions of what my children are saying, what they want of me, and me deciding what it's best to do takes so much energy. It's exhausting.*

Why do those micro-decisions matter so much? The mother just quoted put it simply:

> *We are raising adults.*

These 'avant-garde' mothers (meaning that they are thoughtful individuals, not part of an organised movement) demonstrate the same kind of humanity towards their children that we saw as characteristic of Gaskell. They perceive their children as 'reasonable beings' and 'speak to them kindly.' They tend to have pale, sleep-deprived faces because, in the early years, they respond to their children at night as well as by day. They often talk quietly from exhaustion. Their voices are distinct from the brighter sounds of paid helpers who have more energy. Working with children is tiring, but less so if it's for a limited time. These mothers, however, know they must pace themselves for ongoing hours. It may look like a great sacrifice of their personal time. However, mothers can see a gradual progress in their children's development. They feel rewarded, not financially nor by job advancement, but in the excitement of loving their children, and doing very valuable work for them. As one mother wrote:

> *Loving parents, an open and honest home. It's what I want for my kids. And to help them to become decent people. We have lost sight of how much that matters. I can't think of a more important role* [than a mother bringing up her children]. *And now I'm out and proud enough to say it.*

A mother may find that her child has independent ideas, quite different from her own. He may associate a book with the shape of a screen which is more familiar to him. Screens have a single surface and need to be swiped. One mother was taken aback when she sat down with a book to read to her 10-month-old. But her daughter didn't want the story. The mother finally realised that her daughter wanted to explore the shape of the book, its cover and how to turn its pages. She described what she had learned to a friend:

> First mother: *My daughter wants her own way. I was trying to read her a story, yesterday afternoon, and of course she didn't want to hear it. She wanted to look at the book for herself and turn it at all angles. At first I resisted and tried to continue reading. But then I thought: Why shouldn't she turn the book all over? So I let her.*
>
> Second mother: *I never thought of it like that. My two-year-old still grabs the book when I'm reading to him, and I've always got annoyed with him.*

This is a typical example of the way that mothers learn from one another. The first mother realised that what seemed like 'naughty' behaviour was in reality her daughter's legitimate need to explore. The second mother immediately recognised that this explanation made sense of her son's behaviour too.

Once children can talk, mothers report how amazed they are at their children's original ideas. Given their inexperience, their young thoughts are reasonable. One mother received a surprising 'correction' from her two-year-old:

> *I was reading my daughter a story, when she suddenly interrupted: 'No, Mummy, not like that!' I couldn't think what I was doing wrong. Then she said: 'No, when you turn the pages, you have to lick your fingers first like this.' I had to think about that. I suppose she must have seen a member of staff doing that at her nursery.*

Young children have fine eyes for details, but they have no idea which details are important and which are idiosyncratic. So, at first, as they are novices, they assume that every detail is important, and they connect it to whatever action they are watching. This two-year-old concluded that licking your fingers was essential before turning over the pages of a book. Fortunately, her mother could show her that this was an optional connection and not crucial to reading stories.

Mothers often develop the ability to be still and listen. Children are delighted when their mothers pay attention, and respond, to their ideas. From that, they learn that they matter.

Once a child can talk, he is likely to confront his mother with moral issues. It may be quite a trivial question, such as whether she should allow him to interrupt an adult conversation, or tell him to wait. But serious issues can erupt out of the blue. This happened to one mother:

> *When do you tell the truth? I often want to protect my children from the harsher realities. When my son was two he came back*

> *from nursery and asked: 'What does "kill" mean?' I mean, what do I say?*

The mother knew that the question was important and that her child would register her response. How to reply to a two-year-old needs some thought, even for an experienced mother. She would need to check the context in which her child had heard the word – perhaps another child shouting: 'If you don't come here, I'll kill you!' – and frame her reply in language that her child could understand.

A mother may also discover how sensitive her child is to herself. An example that many will recognise is a time when a mother is facing a difficult situation. Her children, from youngest to oldest, *instantly* pick up on her tension. Just when she is doing her best to cope with the difficult situation itself, her children need her more than ever. One mother said:

> *My husband and I are getting divorced. It's good, but we've got several children, and I'm doing an important job in mothering each of them. I have to be strong. No one else can do this work for me.*

By 'this work' she meant primarily listening to her children and step-children. She was sure that this was important and would make a difference to their lives.

A mother can feel exhausted from trying to understand what her baby is communicating. Perhaps a friend comes round and starts telling her an amusing anecdote. It can feel too much for her. One mother said:

> *I get very tired. I like being in adult company, but when people try telling me about something, say something that happened to them that day, my mind has got too tired to take it in. Sometimes they go on talking, but I find I haven't been listening. There's a whole bit of conversation that I've missed.*

Her friend may not expect this of her either. It isn't widely known. The mother may look as if she is listening by nodding and smiling, but feel inwardly divided between two sorts of conversation, and unable to relax. It surely shows that she is being a good mother, saving her attention for her baby who needs it.

Not all mothers enjoy listening. Some are active women, and see it as their job to teach their children how things work, and how to manage and how to maintain them. They do this by knowing how much their children can understand, and breaking down their teaching into small amounts that their children can manage. They watch their children practising, and teach them the most efficient way.

It's not only their children who are learning. A mother may find herself developing more than she expected. An important quality that has always been associated with mothers is their compassion. They don't seem to be prepared for it, or taught it, and certainly not all mothers practise it. However, one mother, a doctor, said:

> *The main thing I learned from caring for my daughter is compassion. I thought I was compassionate to my patients before. But that was nothing* like *what I felt for them when I returned from my maternity leave.*

Compassion is an ancient concept which has long been associated with mothers. The ancient Hebrew and Arabic terms for it are almost identical: *'rahim'*. The word refers to a womb. The God of the Old Testament unites the properties of male and female, including breasts and a womb. The association of womb with compassion seems to be that the mother's womb generously nurtured her child through pregnancy, and is the source of her divine-like compassion to her child. Later, it spreads outwards to compassion for weak and helpless creatures everywhere. Not all mothers develop compassion, but the quality is often attributed to them.

Many men have awoken to the crucial role of fathers too. Once again, a previously unthinkable revolution has taken place. In many Western countries, fathers are encouraged to be present and assist their partners during the births of their babies. If they can be present at this crucial experience, this helps to give them a sense of their own fatherhood. They may be able to take paternity leave so that they can get to know their newborns properly. They are starting to discover the importance of their unique paternal role. They enjoy being fathers and relating to their children, with all the loving responsibility that this entails.

Mothers with husbands and partners often feel sorry for single mothers, and wonder how they manage. Single mothers report that it can feel endless and very lonely, but there are some advantages. They may not be able to share the parenting with the father, but on the other hand there then is no paternal interference or argument. One single mother reflected when her child was 10 months old:

> *I feel a surge of pride when I look at my daughter. I know I've done all of it by myself. She's filled with a life force, she's joyful and full of wonder.*

Even a mother with a partner often finds herself doing much of the parenting. Despite feminists believing that a mother should share the work equally with her partner, it doesn't always turn out like that. Children have their own ideas. One mother grumbled:

> *There's no equality. My children don't relate to my husband in the same way that they do to me.*

Mothering continues long past childhood. A mother's work has no end. Her child is never 'finished', so neither is her work. Challenging situations continue to arise. Teenagers often turn to their mothers suddenly, and expect them to make time to hear them. Two mothers reflected, independently of one another, on their older children.

> *Babies are easier to satisfy. It's when they are teens that it's hard.*

> *They take a lot from you. They want a lot. It's emotionally very tiring.*
>
> *My daughter's at university and she came home very upset. Her boyfriend had dumped her. I found out that I'm no good at situations like that. I know I should be empathic and just listen to her, but it was very painful for me to hear her.*

In their daily lives, most mothers have been taught as girls that they must stand up for themselves. This marks an important change. Women used to be taught to be deferential, especially to authority. But now mothers study health issues online, collect information for themselves, and are prepared to question doctors, especially, on treatments prescribed for their children. They greatly appreciate doctors who can give them clear explanations. They are not being 'difficult,' as some doctors find them, but taking responsibility for their children. They want to know details of treatments that their parents might simply have accepted without question. Dentists, health visitors, and district nurses come under similar scrutiny.

In print, doctors have lost their monopoly over mothers' health too. For millennia, literature on mothering has been written by doctors. Before the 20th century, they were exclusively men. Some of the advice they gave has been repeated, without evidence, from one medical publication to the next. For example, from ancient Greek times, mothers were advised not to give their babies colostrum, the first food from their breasts.[13] Thanks to La Leche League, which summarised and popularised recent research, we now know that colostrum is *perfect*, both as the first food and also for preparing the newborn's gut for the mother's mature milk, which usually comes in a few days later. But because, for centuries, it used to be considered harmful, babies were given butter or oil, honey or syrup, warmed wine, and other dubious substitutes. 'It's a wonder babies ever survived,' wrote the researcher Valerie Fildes.[14]

Only recently have mothers started to contribute to this

motherhood genre themselves. There are child-centred and mother-centred works. Some are concerned with the practical details of baby care. Others have focused on the very difficult question of how to manage the needs of their babies and themselves. In theory, these works ought to allow for maternal differences and choice. In reality, nearly every book urges mothers to 'do what I've done'. The solutions are nearly always to find ways of surviving in the commercial world.

However, a New Zealand feminist and economist, Marilyn Waring, has pioneered a completely different approach. All around her, she could see women working for their families, for their children and the elderly, tending their livestock and land, if they had any, fetching water, cooking and washing. They worked from morning till night. Without all their work, families couldn't survive. Yet these women lived in poverty. Waring could also see people who did far less essential work, in comfortable offices, and who were well paid.

She did a tremendous amount of research to get to the root of this contradiction, without seeking easy answers. And then she must have seen, suddenly, that the issue was simple. All economies depend on the labour of *women*, she concluded, but the Gross National Product is only calculated by what she defined as male values. She identified these as outcomes that can be measured and sold. A mother's care for her children cannot be measured or sold. So it counts for 'nothing'. Mothers at home, Waring tells us, are considered 'at leisure', or 'unoccupied'. A person caring for *another* woman's baby, feeding the child and baby-sitting, will be thought productive and usually be paid, but a mother doing all of this and more is considered a 'non-producer'.

Waring produced a book with the revealing title: *Counting for Nothing: What Men Value and What Women are Worth*. The title has a double meaning: first, that the act of counting is often pointless, and second that women's unpaid work, such as cleaning and food preparation, cannot be measured or sold, and is therefore seen as worthless.

A much more positive way of measuring production, Waring suggests, is to consider *time*. 'Time is the one thing we all have... Many of us do not trade on the basis of money; we trade our time.'[15] This, she believes, has much more potential to recognise women's work as 'something'. She lists a good deal of the work that mothers do for their families. However, she might also mention all the thinking and planning that precedes the doing. Those take up a lot of a woman's time too.

Waring makes it clear that men calculate production using models that exclude the vital work of women. Women use *time* to produce essential tasks, but the results are ignored as they don't match categories which have market value. Waring's reflections are perceptive, and it must be possible to change the exclusion of women's labours. It would take an economic revolution. Unfortunately, so far, as women, we continue to live in a man's economic world.

One difficulty women face is that the mainstream feminist movement seems to have a negative view of motherhood. New mothers reflect this when they say they dread looking 'mumsy', by which they probably mean looking minimally groomed. Many protest that their bodies have changed, and they can no longer look like their former selves. If they are breastfeeding, their breasts are larger, even for women who once took pride in being flat-chested. Now that they have given birth, they say they want their 'pre-birth bodies back'.

New mothers who do feel proud to have given birth discover that there are few clothes that express their new status. So, if a new mother goes out without her child, there is nothing she can wear to indicate her identity as a mother. Few fashions enhance her motherly appearance. A mother's bodily movements may have become more expansive. In some traditional societies, women indicate their breasts, not to attract men, but to reveal their power. They also wear colourful dresses allowing them to swing their hips, again not to attract men but to express their pleasure in mature womanhood. It is surely significant that few Western mothers appear to have wanted these clothes, nor have dress designers thought it worth exploiting this potential market. What has happened to traditional pride in motherhood?

Yet our female qualities are embodied in us. They contain our potential strength. We obviously can't, and shouldn't, step backwards to return to the frustrated and stereotypical obedient wife, housewife and mother under the patriarchal system that Nightingale abhorred. But we can step forwards.

A number of women who claim that they too are feminists – though they are usually ignored by the mainstream – have tried to show us that women have considerable strengths. I can give two examples of women who taught, published, and encouraged us to enjoy our femininity. Both worked as antenatal teachers. Both discovered the wonders of a woman's body for giving birth, from their own experiences, from research and from teaching. They are Sheila Kitzinger and Janet Balaskas. Both emphasised that a mother's love is more important than doing exercises. So neither is popular with employers, who prefer mothers and babies to be less connected and more easily detached from one another. I am grateful to have been taught by both of them.

The feminist childbirth educator Sheila Kitzinger (1929–2015) is one of these pioneers who have opened up women's sexuality and childbirth in new and exciting ways. As early as the 1950s, she wanted to find a less secretive and much more visible style of being a woman. She found her own way to express her womanhood with flamboyant exuberance. She had enjoyed *giving* birth. The idea of birth as a yielding and giving process was an important concept that she taught. She was one of the founding members of the National Childbirth Trust. In *The Experience of Childbirth*, she encouraged mothers to understand the anatomy of a woman's body and the process of childbirth, and therefore not to fear the various stages but to relax and enjoy them.[16] She was a fiery teacher. 'She spoke truth to power,' recalled her husband, the late international historian, Dr Uwe Kitzinger. 'She never herself sought power – for which those in power must have felt devoutly thankful!'

For example, as an antenatal teacher, she would lie on a stage in front of a large audience, to demonstrate how a woman in labour would look and sound, with loud breathing, sexual moans and bodily gestures, for the different stages. (There's a photo of her doing this on the inside back cover of her autobiography, *A Passion for Birth*.) Many women have said that they found this liberating as well as educational.

Kitzinger's first degree was in social anthropology, and this became very useful to her. She travelled widely, and discussed childbirth with women from different cultures. On one journey, she visited Turkish carpet-sellers, and made an exciting discovery. 'Freud introduced us to phallic symbols,' she wrote. 'The symbol of women's life-giving energy, however, remained mostly hidden and mysterious. Yet they were all around us in textiles made by women in countries stretching from the Middle East to the Pacific.'[17]

> *Throughout history and even in prehistory, in many different cultures the concept of the life-giving vagina has been an important symbolic motif in women's weaving and other crafts. Men have usually not known what it meant. The birth symbol takes the form of a hooked diamond, sometimes with a cross representing the fetus inside of the diamond. There are 17 structurally distinct variations on this basic theme which appear on artefacts made by women in cultures all over the world. They can often be discovered for example, in traditional rugs and wall-hangings woven by women. The sign represents both vagina and uterus and is the counterpart of the male phallic symbol.*[18]

'The life-giving vagina' – how many women think of their vaginas like that? Kitzinger was fascinated to discover so many examples. Men generally sold the beautiful rugs and wall-hangings, so Kitzinger would ask them if they knew what these symbols were. But they couldn't give her satisfactory answers. The women who wove them were aware of what they meant. Even when she and they didn't have a common language, they were able to point to one another's bodies, and understand one another, to their mutual delight.

Her book *A Celebration of Birth* contains 28 pages of Kitzinger's poems and paintings. She had spent decades in teaching and writing to guide midwives, and to help and comfort women who had more difficult births than her own. In *A Celebration of Birth,* she finally gave voice to her own experiences. She wasn't teaching, and obviously didn't expect any pregnant mother to believe she was meant to copy her. So her poems are honest and intimate. Each is beautifully expressed, so I've chosen one example. The punctuation is exactly as printed.

> *Birth is power.*
> *Not frail and fancy suffering*
> *not a passive waiting on life*
> *not polite obedience to medical commands or coaxing.*
> *The cloud burst.*
> *Woman arches over all*
> *queen of the night, goddess of creation*
> *in splendour and strength of majesty.*
> *The tempest of life's beginning*
> *sweeps through her body.*
> *The flower opens.*
> *Thick petals part.*
> *The hard bud pushes down*
> *and spreads wide*
> *tissues that burn with sacred fire.*[19]

Kitzinger knew that many women had been told dreadful accounts of painful births by their families or friends, and approached their own births with dread. She did not. She had five daughters, including a pair of twins. 'There is *nothing* to fear about childbirth,' she would say, which was evidently true of her own experience. Because she was not afraid, she experienced the wonderful strength of her female body, and realised that it was perfectly designed to give birth. Women only needed, she taught, to let go of fear.

My labours were not ecstatic. However, there are many accounts by other women who discovered the wonder of childbirth. So Kitzinger's experiences were individual but not unique.

She also described life after childbirth, and how most mothers enjoyed relating intimately to their babies. But she knew other mothers who were advised to respond differently.

> *Advice is given to the mother to 'show the baby who is master,'* [Note the male image.] *'Let him see you are in command.' But these are extraordinary words to use about this most tender and subtle form of human relationships, and hardly form an adequate response to the child's need for his mother, and his adoration of her.*[20]

I attended two of her classes before the birth of my first child, and then telephoned to explain that I couldn't come to the third. While we were talking, my very strong birth contractions started suddenly, and she was wonderfully supportive. 'Your breathing is beautifully rhythmical,' she assured me. She wrote that she always found something positive to say to a labouring woman, even if it was: 'What a lovely frock you're wearing.' She stayed on the phone until my husband joined me 'because you shouldn't be alone.' Then she said we should ring for an ambulance and go to hospital. I felt bereft of her comforting presence when she rang off.

Another pioneering childbirth educator is Janet Balaskas, who originally trained at one of Kitzinger's National Childbirth Trust classes in London. One early discovery that Balaskas made was that women's bodies were not 'made' to give birth flat on their backs or semi-reclining, as often happens on hospital beds even now. Historical evidence in art showed women giving birth in upright positions, on birth stools, kneeling or squatting. So this was what she taught. She soon realised that many modern women had stiff muscles. They had spent years of sedentary life at school desks, and after that at their jobs. Many expectant mothers continue to work until their first birth contractions begin. They need preparation for a good birth experience. So Balaskas devised a programme of wonderful yoga-based exercises to loosen women's muscles. Pregnancy was the ideal time to learn them, she said, because a pregnant woman's body was preparing for birth and becoming more flexible anyway. Balaskas said she believed that her yoga-based exercises could enable a woman of any age and level of stiffness to soften her muscles and be able to squat.

I attended her classes before the birth of my third child, and she was right. I had just turned 40, and was surprised at my own confidence in the new flexibility of my body. I looked forward to giving birth. This was fortunate as my third baby, born at home, was a 'brow presentation'. My experienced obstetrician was puzzled that the last stage of the birth was taking so long, and called out the Flying Squad (a team that was then available to rush to the bedside of a labouring mother in an emergency). But I remained calm. I could feel the baby suddenly start to move downwards inside me and, to my relief, was able to give birth normally, so the Flying Squad had to be turned back. The obstetrician asked me to hand the baby to him to check, and exclaimed: 'Ah, you have a red mark across your brow, you were a *brow* presentation. I haven't seen one of those for decades. Well, you gave us a fright, young man!' But, thanks to Balaskas's classes, I hadn't been frightened, and was delighted to hold my third child in my arms at last.

Balaskas was clear that medical advances 'undoubtedly save lives', and are important for times when a birth is complicated.

> *Yet, as a result of the indiscriminate and widespread application of these* [medical] *interventions... many women today have lost faith in their innate ability to give birth unaided. They approach the experience with fear, anticipating pain and complications. ...Ironically the anxiety* [that] *this may cause leads women to produce stress hormones that can inhibit and delay the normal onset of labour.*[21]

She demonstrated in her classes, with a model pelvis and a doll, that a woman's body is uniquely designed to give birth to a baby in an upright position, in harmony with gravity, especially when women are given the freedom to keep changing position as the baby descends. In case this sounds like hard work:

> *Women's bodies are designed to produce high levels of ecstatic birth hormones, which help us to enjoy giving birth and also to love and mother our babies.*[22]

At the end of each exercise class, Balaskas would invite the expectant mothers to lie back on the floor, relax, and see if they could contact their babies. Here may be one reason why mainstream feminists do not favour these childbirth classes. Both Kitzinger and Balaskas spoke warmly about the maternal relationship, and encouraged mothers to feel connected to their babies from the start. So these mother-and-baby couples are likely to become mutually loving and attached. This might make it much more difficult for them to separate, conveniently, at the end of maternity leave. Separation of mother and baby may be good for a woman's career, but can't do justice to the needs of a loving mother-and-baby couple.

Another exciting issue for mothers is breastfeeding. There are written instructions on how to do it, but breastfeeding seems to work best when it is visual and a mother has sat together with a number of breastfeeding women. She can then see that each woman's body is a different shape, and also the shapes of their breasts and even their areolae and nipples vary too. All these breasts are producing milk. There can't possibly be only one 'correct' position or one way to hold the baby that is exactly the same for everyone. Watching several mothers breastfeeding is a good way to learn, because the eye selects visual cues quicker than the mother's mind can formulate verbal rules. It's interesting that, when a mother is breastfeeding in a park, little children of five and under, boys as well as girls, often come and watch. Perhaps what they observe is stored in a 'memory bank' to help them when their time comes.

Many mothers say they have tried hard but have failed to produce enough breastmilk. With the help of an experienced and supportive mother, most women can learn how. Unfortunately, many have grown up watching mothers bottle-feeding. This puts the mother in charge. She holds the bottle and angles it towards her baby's mouth. But breastfeeding empowers the baby. It's the baby who has to angle his head in the right position. He then opens his mouth and dives onto the breast. His mother needs to sit in a good position, but cannot do the 'fine tuning' for him. She is looking down at him, whereas his viewpoint is more accurate, lying parallel to her breasts.

Relaxation is the key. I used to be a La Leche League leader, and I remember making a home visit to a mother who was in despair at not being able to breastfeed. She had large breasts, so getting her into a good position took time. 'I can't do it. My baby's lost interest,' she wailed. So we started chatting about something different. Suddenly, she whispered: *'Look!'* While we'd stopped trying, her baby suddenly noticed what a good position she was in, and latched on beautifully. She got her husband to come in and take photographs, so that she could help her baby to do it again.

Thanks to La Leche League, the international breastfeeding charity, we now know that breastmilk is unique and that even expressing it and feeding the baby with a bottle is not quite the same. The mother produces breastmilk in an ideal digestible sequence for her baby. Her milk also keeps pace with her baby's growth and development so that, at two years, her milk has adapted and is not the same as when her baby was newborn.[23]

La Leche League wants to be 'inclusive', and has started calling breastmilk 'human milk'. But this is not the same. It's the *mother's* milk that the baby needs most. That was the original foundation of La Leche League's philosophy.

Anyone who has only seen mothers struggling to breastfeed would be amazed to see how wonderful it looks when mother and baby have discovered how. These babies often want to continue breastfeeding well into toddlerhood. It's a joyful experience. They crow with delight, pat their mothers' breasts, and their mothers look delighted. Many mothers have overcome early difficulties such as the baby's tongue-tie or her mastitis to get to this point. Journals published by La Leche League contain stories and photos that illustrate just how wonderful an experience it can be. Mother and child have formed a tender relationship, through breastfeeding and also through their bodily closeness.

A loving approach to childbirth, and breastfeeding, provides truly feminine, emotional and embodied introductions to motherhood. It's not easy for a woman today to make the transition from a male-orientated environment straight into the heart of a female one. Works by Sheila Kitzinger and Janet Balaskas, and La Leche League's book *The Art of Breastfeeding*, contain practical information, together with loving, spiritual qualities, which honour both mother and baby. These can guide new mothers as they enter an unfamiliar culture. In my earlier books, especially the first – *What Mothers Do: especially when it looks like nothing* – I quote mothers talking in their own words about the lack of existing vocabulary to describe what it is that mothers do.

Many books, conferences, and workshops end with vehement calls to the government to make conditions easier for mothers, and for society to change. But mothers haven't made a strong enough case for what we achieve to have an impact on our society and the government. Besides, we are a large proportion of society. If we are able to see motherhood positively, we can reverse the prevailing social negativity.

Why is it always up to *others* to instigate change on behalf of mothers?

Only we, as mothers, understand how much we are contributing to social life. Do we need to use apologetic language to refer to ourselves as 'only mothers' who perhaps have taken 'too much time off' for maternity leave? Perhaps it is up to grandmothers to speak up for mothers. Looking back, many of us can see the situation clearly. We surely sympathise with the dilemma of this mother:

> *I'm living on the edge all the time, constantly thinking about money, waking at three in the morning, thinking about debt, overthinking every decision. My middle child is very athletic and wanted to do kickboxing classes, but they're £11.50 a time. I told her: 'We can't.' They're really good kids. They understand.*[24]

'Really good kids' don't drop down from the sky. They are nurtured, day and night, in this case by a caring mother. There ought to be a way of enabling generous mothering to count, not only in time, but in *quality*. There should be a way of relieving this mother's invaluable work from financial stress.

What we need is not an immediate financial solution for the Gaskells of our society, but a change in the pervasive attitude towards mothers. Many of our achievements have no words to identify them, so it's difficult for us to see them ourselves. That lack of language is part of our challenge. The more we can appreciate ourselves as mothers, the better we can present ourselves. We should not be beggars. We should not have to grovel for financial help. We have gathered a wide range of experience. Each of us is a vital component of our civilisation.

Towards the end of *Cassandra*, Nightingale wrote: 'Awake, ye women, all ye that sleep, awake!'[25] She was a committed Christian and studied her Bible in detail, verse by verse. She annotated almost every chapter of the book of the Hebrew prophet Isaiah[26] who first used the double 'Awake, awake'.[27] These words have been repeated since, but they must have sounded revolutionary when Isaiah first thought of them. He saw that waking up could mean not only waking from sleep, but also from a state of despairing torpor. It's exciting to look back and recognise that women really have awoken to Nightingale's revolutionary call.

Surely it's as *mothers* that we women are 'asleep' today. Just as Nightingale saw that the majority of women were comfortably sleeping in their servitude to their husbands, so now many mothers believe they are liberated, while in reality they seem caught in servitude to the economic systems of Western society. Many feel unhappy and guilty for seeing so little of their children, but can't see an alternative.

We can't move on without adjusting the social pendulum. We need a radically new attitude towards motherhood. This is a vital way *forward*, not back. In a period of declining birthrates, mothers who long to give their energies to their children should have the means to do so.

Certainly women differ. Some don't want children, while others want children but prefer to combine mothering with their careers. There is no single mould for every woman. Some are natural Nightingales, others Gaskells, while many of us are a mixture of both. All are contributing to a dynamic society.

The 'grand quarrel' made sense in 1845. Today we are in a position to resolve it. We need our Nightingales. But why should we snub our Gaskells? Nightingale's original view was expressed in the fighting words that Gaskell reported: 'If she [Nightingale] had influence enough not a mother should bring up a child herself.' Now this has become almost a reality. Why? Is this what every mother wants?

'Awake, awake!'

Can we mothers *wake up* to appreciate what wonderful work we do? Dare we recognise our true worth?

With thanks

To all those mothers who trusted me and have talked and written to me. To editor, Anne Newman; my daughter Rachel Stadlen; and my husband, Anthony Stadlen, who read and made such excellent comments and corrections on every chapter of early versions of *A Grand Quarrel*. To the Motherhood Initiative for Research and Community Involvement who first heard 'A Grand Quarrel' given as a short talk in Athens in April 2014, and to the Elizabeth Gaskell House for enabling me to give a longer version on Zoom, during the lockdown period, in November 2020. To Peter Kay, then owner of Lea Hurst, for responding to my questions. To Sonya Moudart and Siân Morgan who read chapters. To my wonderful family, my children: Rachel, Shoël and Darrel, and to my grandchildren: Tovi, Anya and Antoshka, and to my loving husband who was close to tears when *A Grand Quarrel* was accepted and understood by a publisher at last.

To Martin Wagner, publisher, who saw the importance of this work, and to Susan Last, who lives near Lea Hurst, for editing it.

Bibliography

Athan, Aurélie A. and Miller, Lisa (2013) 'Motherhood as opportunity to learn spiritual values: experience and insights of new mothers' in *Journal of Prenatal and Perinatal Psychology and Health*, 27(4), summer 2013

Austen, Jane (1816) *Emma*. Many editions

Balaskas, Janet (2023) *Active Birth*, London: Pinter & Martin

Barnett, Emma (2025) *Maternity Leave/Service*. London: Fig Tree/Penguin Books

Brown, Solveig (2014) 'Intensive mothering as an adaptive response' in Ennis, Linda Rose, ed. *Intensive Mothering*. Bradford, Ontario: Demeter Press

Chapple, J.A.V. (1980) *Elizabeth Gaskell: A portrait in letters*. Manchester: Manchester University Press

Chapple, John (1997) *Elizabeth Gaskell: the early years*. Manchester: Manchester University Press

Chapple, J.A.V. and Pollard, Arthur, eds. (1966) *The Letters of Mrs Gaskell*. Manchester: Manchester University Press

Chapple, John and Shelston, Alan, eds. (2000) *Further Letters of Mrs Gaskell*. Manchester: Manchester University Press

Chapple, J.A.V. and Wilson, Anita, eds. (1996) *Private Voices, the Diaries of Elizabeth Gaskell and Sophie Holland*. Keele: Keele University Press

Cook, E. (1914) *The Life of Florence Nightingale*. London: Macmillan

Cromwell, Judith Lissauer (2013) *Florence Nightingale, Feminist*. Jefferson, North Carolina: McFarland

Dexter, Walter, ed. (1938) *The Letters of Charles Dickens*. Bloomsbury: The Nonesuch Press

Eliot, G. (1871-72) *Middlemarch*. Many editions

Gaskell, E.C. (1848) *Mary Barton*. Many editions

Gaskell, E.C. (1853a) *Cranford*. Many editions

Gaskell, E.C. (1853b) *Ruth*. Many editions

Gaskell, E.C. (1855) *North and South*. Many editions

Gaskell, E.C. (1997 [1857]) *The Life of Charlotte Bronte*. London: Penguin

Gaskell, E.C. (1866) *Wives and Daughters*. Many editions

Gérin, Winifred (1976) *Elizabeth Gaskell*. Oxford: Oxford University Press

Gill, Gillian (2004) *Nightingales, Florence and her Family*. London: Hodder & Stoughton

Haldane, Elizabeth (1930) *Mrs Gaskell and Her Friends*. London: Hodder & Stoughton

Hamilton, Edith and Cairns, Huntington, eds. (1961) *The Collected Dialogues of Plato*. New York: Bollingen Foundation

Hewitt, Llewellyn (1855) *A Stroll to Lea Hurst, Derbyshire Home of Florence Nightingale*. London. This piece first appeared in the *Derby Telegraph* in May 1855, and then as a booklet, priced threepence. A copy is held in the

British Library.
Hicks, Jennifer, ed. (2006) *Hirkani's Daughters*. Schaumburg, Illinois: La Leche League International
Janacek Reeber, Brianne and Caplan, Paula J. (2014) 'Are "Mommy Wars" real?' in Reid Boyd, Elizabeth and Letherby, Gale, eds. (2014) *Stay-at-Home Mothers*. Bradford, Ontario: Demeter Press
Jones, Lucy (2023) *Matrescence*. London: Allen Lane
Kitzinger, Sheila (1967) *The Experience of Childbirth*. London: Victor Gollancz
Kitzinger, Sheila (1986) *A Celebration of Birth*. Seattle, Washington: Pennypress
Kitzinger, Sheila (2015) *A Passion for Birth*. London: Pinter & Martin
Locke, John (1689-90) *An Essay Concerning Human Understanding*. Many editions
Lohrli, Anne, comp. (1973) *Household Words, A weekly journal 1850-59*. Toronto: University of Toronto Press
McDonald, Lynn, ed. (2001–12) *The Collected Works of Florence Nightingale*. Waterloo, Ontario: Wilfrid Laurier University Press
Maxwell, J.C., ed. (1971) *William Wordsworth, The Prelude, a parallel text*. London: Penguin
Nightingale, Florence (1979) *Cassandra*. Old Westbury, New York: The Feminist Press
Nightingale, Florence (1861) *Notes on Nursing for the Labouring Classes*. London: Harrison
O'Malley, I.B. (1931) *Florence Nightingale*. London: Thornton, Butterworth
Osborne, Lord Sidney Godolphin (1855) *Scutari and its hospitals*. London: Dickenson
Reid Boyd, Elizabeth and Letherby, Gale, eds. (2014) *Stay-at-Home Mothers*. Bradford, Ontario: Demeter Press
Sanders, Valerie, ed. (1990) *Harriet Martineau, Selected Letters*. Oxford: Clarendon Press
Shore, Tricia (2006) 'A funny thing happened...' in Hicks, Jennifer, ed. (2006) *Hirkani's Daughters*. Schaumburg, Illinois: La Leche League International
Temkin, Owsei, trans. (1956) *Soranus' Gynecology*. Baltimore: John Hopkins University Press
Uglow, Jenny (1993) *Elizabeth Gaskell*. London: Faber and Faber
Ulbrich, Tara (2014) 'Motherhood as an act of personal and social co-creation' in Reid Boyd, Elizabeth and Letherby, Gale, eds. (2014) *Stay-at-Home Mothers*. Bradford, Ontario: Demeter Press
Verney, Lady Frances Parthenope (1855?) *Life and Death of Athena, an owlet from the Parthenon*.
Vicinus, Martha and Nergaard, Bea, eds. (1990) *Ever Yours, Florence Nightingale: Selected Letters*. Cambridge, Massachusetts: Harvard University Press
Waring, Marilyn (1999) *Counting for Nothing: What Men Value and What Women are Worth*. Toronto: University of Toronto Press
Wiessinger, Diane; West, Diana; and Pitman, Teresa for La Leche League International (2010) *The Womanly Art of Breastfeeding*. London: Pinter & Martin

Notes

Introduction

1. Chapple (1980). The quotation from the quarrel is on page xii.

References to Elizabeth Gaskell's letters are to the letter number followed by the page number on which the letter starts.

Chapter 1: A Visit to Lea Hurst

1. Haldane (1930), p.288.
2. Hewitt (1855), p.21.
3. Hewitt (1855), pp.23-24.
4. Hewitt (1855), p.8.
5. Hewitt (1855), p.13.
6. Hewitt (1855), p.18.
7. Chapple and Pollard (1966), letter 218, p.321.
8. McDonald (2002), Vol. 1, p.414.
9. Chapple and Pollard (1966), letter 444, p.579.
10. Chapple and Pollard (1966), letter 216, p.315.
11. Chapple and Pollard (1966), letter 211, p.305. William Whewell (1794–1866), a brilliant English polymath, had written *On the Plurality of Worlds* (1853), claiming to refute the idea that there was life on other planets.
12. Chapple and Pollard (1966), letter 211, p.305.
13. Chapple and Pollard (1966), letter 211, p.305.
14. Chapple and Pollard (1966), letter 515, p.693.
15. Chapple and Pollard (1966), letter 211, p.305.
16. Chapple (1997), p.118.
17. These two passages are from Gaskell (1853a), Chapter 5.
18. Chapple and Pollard (1966), letter 212, p.310.
19. Chapple and Pollard (1966), letter 211, p.305.

Chapter 2: Parthenope: 'Athena, an owlet from the Parthenon'

1. Verney (1855?)
2. Chapple and Pollard (1966), letter 215, p.314.
3. Vicinus and Nergaard (1990), pp.110-111.

Chapter 3: Gaskell: 'I feel myself so unknowing'

1. Chapple and Wilson (1996), p.121.
2. Chapple (1997), p.437.
3. Uglow (1993), p.11.
4. For the unnamed son, see Chapple and Shelston (2000), p.156.

5. The birth dates of Gaskell's children are:
   Her stillborn daughter, July 1833;
   Marianne, 12 September 1834;
   Meta, 5 February 1837;
   An unnamed son (see previous note);
   Florence, 7 October 1842;
   Willie, 23 October 1844–10 August 1845; and
   Julia, 3 September 1846.
6. Austen (1816), Chapter 1
7. Maxwell (1971), lines 237-243.
8. Chapple and Pollard (1966), letter 12, p.28.
9. Chapple and Pollard (1966), letter 614, p.796.
10. Gaskell (1866), Chapter 1.
11. Chapple (1980), p.5.
12. Chapple (1997), p.223.
13. Gaskell (1855), Chapter 14.
14. Chapple (1997), p.338.
15. Chapple and Pollard (1966), letter 12, p.28.
16. See Lohrli (1973). Also Gérin (1976), p.261.
17. Uglow (1993), p.95.
18. Chapple and Wilson (1996), p.50.
19. Chapple and Wilson (1996), p.53.
20. Chapple and Wilson (1996), p.50.
21. Chapple and Wilson (1996), p.53.
22. Chapple and Wilson (1996), p.121.
23. Chapple and Wilson (1996), p.50.
24. Athan and Miller (2013)
25. Chapple and Wilson (1996), p.53.
26. Chapple and Wilson (1996), p.61.
27. Chapple and Wilson (1996), p.50.
28. Chapple and Wilson (1996), p.51.
29. Gaskell (1997 [1857]), p.127.
30. Chapple and Wilson (1996), p.51.
31. Chapple and Wilson (1996), p.58.
32. Chapple and Wilson (1996), p.58.
33. Chapple and Wilson (1996), p.51.
34. Locke (1689-90), Essay I, iv, 2.
35. Chapple and Wilson (1996), p.51.
36. Chapple and Wilson (1996), p.51.
37. Albertine Adrienne Necker de Saussure (1766-1841). 'The tears of children are so bitter, the perfect calm of the soul is so necessary to them that tears must above all be spared.'
38. Chapple and Wilson (1996), p.52.
39. Chapple and Wilson (1996), p.54.

40. Chapple and Wilson (1996), p.52.
41. Chapple and Wilson (1996), p.56.
42. Chapple and Wilson (1996), p.57.
43. Chapple and Wilson (1996), p.58.
44. Chapple and Wilson (1996), p.54.
45. Chapple and Wilson (1996), p.61.
46. Chapple and Wilson (1996), p.68.
47. Chapple and Wilson (1996), p.63.
48. Chapple and Wilson (1996), p.65.
49. Chapple and Wilson (1996), p.62.
50. Chapple and Wilson (1996), p.69.
51. Chapple and Wilson (1996), p.65.
52. Chapple and Wilson (1996), p.66.
53. Chapple and Pollard (1966), letter 453, p.597.
54. Chapple and Pollard (1966), letter 214, p.313.
55. Chapple and Pollard (1966), letter 68, p.106.
56. Chapple and Pollard (1966), letter 515, p.693.

Chapter 4: Gaskell: 'If I could get over this next piece'

1. McDonald (2001–12), Vol. 5, p.785.
2. Chapple and Pollard (1966), letter 150, p.222.
3. Dexter (1938), Vol. II, p.202.
4. Dexter (1938), Vol. II, p.364.
5. Chapple and Pollard (1966), letter 153, p.226.
6. Chapple and Pollard (1966), letter 36, p.67.
7. Dexter (1938), Vol. II, pp.561-562.
8. Dexter (1938), Vol. II, p.570.
9. Dexter (1938), Vol. II, p.598.
10. Chapple and Shelston (2000), p.227.
11. Chapple and Pollard (1966), letter 211, p.305.
12. Gaskell (1855), Chapter 19.
13. Gaskell (1855), Chapter 20.
14. Gaskell (1855), Chapter 25.
15. Gaskell (1855), Chapter 26.
16. Chapple and Pollard (1966), letter 217, p.316.
17. Chapple and Pollard (1966), letter 225, p.328.
18. Chapple and Pollard (1966), letter 220, p.323.
19. Chapple and Pollard (1966), letter 227, p.330.
20. Haldane (1930), p.113.
21. Haldane (1930), p.114. Also Chapple and Pollard (1966), letter 223, p.327.
22. Chapple and Pollard (1966), letter 217, p.315.
23. Chapple and Pollard (1966), letter 211, p.305.
24. Chapple and Pollard (1966), letter 218, p.321.
25. Chapple and Pollard (1966), letter 217, p.315.

26. Chapple and Pollard (1966), letter 217, p.316.
27. Chapple and Pollard (1966), letter 218, p.321.
28. Chapple and Pollard (1966), letter 218, p.321.
29. Chapple and Pollard (1966), letter 228, p.331.
30. Chapple and Pollard (1966), letter 215, p.314.

Chapter 5: Nightingale: 'I have no desire now but to die'

Vicinus and Nergaard (1990), p.54.
2. Vicinus and Nergaard (1990), p.46.
3. Vicinus and Nergaard (1990), p.46.
4. Vicinus and Nergaard (1990), p.47.
5. O'Malley (1931), p.15.
6. Cromwell (2013), p.15.
7. Chapple and Pollard (1966), letter 217, p.316.
8. Chapple and Pollard (1966), letter 217, p.316.
9. Chapple and Pollard (1966), letter 211, p.305.
10. Nightingale (1979), p.30.
11. Chapple and Pollard (1966), letter 211, p.305.
12. Gill (2004), p.448.
13. Cromwell (2013), p.9.
14. Vicinus and Nergaard (1990), p.29.
15. McDonald (2001–12), Vol. 1, p.830.
16. 'Notes on the Family' in McDonald (2001–12), Vol. 5, p.236.
17. Chapple and Pollard (1966), letter 217, p.316.
18. Vicinus and Nergaard (1990), p.36.
19. McDonald (2001–12), Vol. 11, p.25.
20. Cromwell (2013), p.39.
21. O'Malley (1931), pp.26-27.
22. Vicinus and Nergaard (1990), p.45.
23. 'Notes on the Family' in McDonald (2001–12), Vol. 5, p.233.
24. Vicinus and Nergaard (1990), p.44.
25. 'Notes on the Family' in McDonald (2001–12), Vol. 5, p.233.
26. Vicinus and Nergaard (1990), pp.60-61.
27. Vicinus and Nergaard (1990), p.47.
28. Nightingale (1979), p.25.
29. Nightingale (1979), p.25.
30. Nightingale (1979), p.29.
31. Nightingale (1979), p.30.
32. Nightingale (1979), p.33.
33. Nightingale (1979), p.34.
34. Vicinus and Nergaard (1990), p.46.
35. Chapple and Pollard (1966), letter 217, p.316.
36. Nightingale (1979), p. 37.
37. Vicinus and Nergaard (1990), pp.47 and 50.

38. McDonald (2001–12), Vol. 3, p.152.
39. Nightingale (1979), p.38.
40. Nightingale (1979), p.28.
41. Nightingale (1979), p.40.
42. Nightingale (1979), p.41.
43. Nightingale (1979), p.52.
44. Nightingale (1979), p.53.
45. Nightingale (1979), pp.54-55.

Chapter 6: Nightingale: 'No one will act but me'

1. Vicinus and Nergaard (1990), p.44.
2. Vicinus and Nergaard (1990), pp.48 and 60.
3. Vicinus and Nergaard (1990), p.49.
4. Vicinus and Nergaard (1990), p.60.
5. Vicinus and Nergaard (1990), p.63.
6. McDonald (2001–12), Vol. 5, p.234.
7. Chapple and Pollard (1966), letter 217, p.317.
8. Chapple and Pollard (1966), letter 217, p.317.
9. O'Malley (1931), p.199.
10. Vicinus and Nergaard (1990), p.67.
11. Chapple and Pollard (1966), letter 211, p.305.
12. Chapple and Pollard (1966), letter 217, p.316.
13. Chapple and Pollard (1966), letter 217, p.316.
14. McDonald (2001–12), Vol. 1, p.317.
15. Chapple and Pollard (1966), letter 211, p.305.
16. Chapple and Pollard (1966), letter 211, p.305.
17. Chapple and Pollard (1966), letter 150, p.222.
18. Chapple and Pollard (1966), letter 217, p.316.
19. Chapple and Pollard (1966), letter 217, p.316.
20. McDonald (2001–12), Vol. 1, p.65. From a letter to her father dated 12 October 1867.
21. McDonald (2001–12), Vol. 1, pp.80-81.
22. Chapple and Pollard (1966), letter 217, p.320
23. McDonald (2001–12), Vol. 14, p.55.
24. McDonald (2001–12), Vol. 14, p.47. A copy of Sir Sidney Herbert's letter, dated 15 October 1854, is in the Verney Collection 10/319/34.
25. McDonald (2001–12), Vol. 14, p.55.
26. Vicinus and Nergaard (1990), p.79.
27. Vicinus and Nergaard (1990), p.48.
28. 'Notes on the family' in McDonald (2001–12), Vol. 5, p.232.

Chapter 7: Gaskell: 'A grand quarrel'

1. Gaskell (1848), Preface.

2. Gaskell (1848), Chapter 15.
3. Vicinus and Nergaard (1990), p.148.
4. Vicinus and Nergaard (1990), p.158.
5. McDonald (2001–12), Vol. 15, p.37.
6. Nightingale (1861), Preface and p.10.
7. Chapple and Pollard (1966), letter 68, p.106.
8. Chapple and Pollard (1966), letter 39, p.69.
9. McDonald (2001–12), Vol. 1, p.24.
10. Chapple and Pollard (1966), letter 69, p.107.
11. Gaskell (1853b), Chapter 14.
12. Gaskell (1853b), Chapter 31.
13. Chapple and Pollard (1966), letter 349, p.450.
14. Nightingale (1979), p.36.
15. Nightingale (1979), p.42. In her biography of Elizabeth Gaskell, Jenny Uglow describes Gaskell's similar irritation. 'Her idea of social misery was a stuffy dinner party or a "grave and serious" tea of the kind she described in "Company Manners" in 1854. At this tea-party, the talk was as heavy as the food, and in every ponderous silence the hostess would say, "eat another macaroon."' Uglow (1993), p.237.
16. Haldane (1930), pp.288-289.
17. Chapple and Pollard (1966), letter 409, p.524.
18. Chapple and Pollard (1966), letter 420, p.542.
19. Chapple and Pollard (1966), letter 171, p.255.
20. Eliot (1871-72), Chapter 12.
21. Chapple and Pollard (1966), letter 217, p.316.
22. McDonald (2001–12), Vol. 11, p.441.
23. McDonald (2001–12), Vol. 1, p.219. From a letter to William Nightingale dated 18 December 1827.
24. McDonald (2001–12), Vol. 11, p.352.
25. Hamilton and Cairns (1961), Book V, p.694.
26. Hamilton and Cairns (1961), Book V, pp.694-695.
27. Nightingale (1979), p.37.
28. Hamilton and Cairns (1961), Book V, p.699.
29. McDonald (2001–12), Vol. 5, p.602. This and the next quotation come from her comments on Benjamin Jowett's second edition of *Dialogues of Plato* (1875). Nightingale corrected it in detail, line by line. Jowett said he had used nearly all her suggestions and felt hugely indebted to her. 'You are the best critic I have ever had,' he told her. (See E. Cook [1914], *The Life of Florence Nightingale*. London: Macmillan, Vol. 2, p.225.)
30. McDonald (2001–12), Vol. 5, p.602.

Chapter 8: Gaskell: 'Or will you snub me?'

1. McDonald (2001–12), Vol. 14, p.180.
2. Chapple and Pollard (1966), letter 218, p.321.

3. Chapple and Pollard (1966), letter 236, p.341.
4. McDonald (2001–12), Vol. 1, p.33.
5. McDonald (2001–12), Vol. 14, p.211.
6. McDonald (2001–12), Vol. 14, p.62.
7. McDonald (2001–12), Vol. 14, p.758.
8. Osborne (1855), p.26.
9. Osborne (1855), p.24.
10. McDonald (2001–12), Vol. 8, p.56.
11. Chapple and Pollard (1966), letter 262, p.366.
12. Chapple and Pollard (1966), letter 268, p.370.
13. Chapple and Pollard (1966), letter 279, p.382.
14. Chapple and Pollard (1966), letter 279, p.382.
15. Chapple and Pollard (1966), letter 300, p.402.
16. Chapple and Pollard (1966), letter 217, p.316.
17. McDonald (2001–12), Vol. 1, p.30.
18. Chapple and Pollard (1966), letter 40, p.71.
19. McDonald (2001–12), Vol. 14, p.991.
20. McDonald (2001–12), Vol. 14, p.793.
21. McDonald (2001–12), Vol. 14, p.791.
22. McDonald (2001–12), Vol. 14, p.647.
23. McDonald (2001–12), Vol. 14, p.981.
24. McDonald (2001–12), Vol. 14, p.204.
25. McDonald (2001–12), Vol. 14, p.828.
26. McDonald (2001–12), Vol. 8, pp.110ff.
27. McDonald (2001–12), Vol. 14, p.993.
28. Sanders (1990), pp.166ff.
29. McDonald (2001–12), Vol. 14, p.993.
30. McDonald (2001–12), Vol. 14, p.990.
31. Chapple and Shelston (2000), pp.192-193.
32. McDonald (2001–12), Vol. 5, p.785.
33. McDonald (2001–12), Vol. 5, p.781.
34. McDonald (2001–12), Vol. 15, p.433.
35. McDonald (2001–12), Vol. 8, p.814. The original is in the John Rylands Library, Manchester University, ENG MS 731.
36. Chapple and Shelston (2000), p.257.
37. Chapple and Pollard (1966), letter 583, pp.773.
38. Chapple and Shelston (2000), p.266.
39. Chapple and Pollard (1966), letter 561, p.746.
40. Chapple and Pollard (1966), letter 565, p.751.
41. Chapple and Pollard (1966), letter 575a, p.936.
42. Chapple and Pollard (1966), letter 582b, p.940.
43. Chapple and Pollard (1966), letter 582, p.771.
44. McDonald (2001–12), Vol. 1, p.536. The letter is dated 1845, but this must be a misprint for 1865.

45. McDonald (2001–12), Vol. 3, pp.143-144.
46. McDonald (2001–12), Vol. 5, p.602.
47. McDonald (2001–12), Vol. 1, p.15. The contract is dated 1 July 1820.
48. McDonald (2001–12), Vol. 5, p.603.
49. Vicinus and Nergaard (1990), p.178.
50. Vicinus and Nergaard (1990), p.171.
51. Vicinus and Nergaard (1990), pp.164-165.
52. McDonald (2001–12), Vol. 1, p.54.

Chapter 9: Nightingale: 'Treat them like reasonable beings'

1. McDonald (2001–12), Vol.1, p.65. From a letter to William Nightingale dated 12 October 1867.
2. Vicinus and Nergaard (1990), p.432.
3. Osborne (1855), p.46.
4. Chapple and Pollard (1966), letter 255, p.358. '[F]or we have all of us one human heart' is quoted from the poem 'The Old Cumberland Beggar' by William Wordsworth.
5. McDonald (2001–12), Vol. 1, p.93.
6. Vicinus and Nergaard (1990), p.56.
7. McDonald (2001–12), Vol. 1, p.92.
8. McDonald (2001–12), Vol. 1, p.91.
9. Vicinus and Nergaard (1990), p.47.
10. Vicinus and Nergaard (1990), p.50.
11. Vicinus and Nergaard (1990), p.52.
12. Chapple and Pollard (1966), letter 211, p.305.
13. Vicinus and Nergaard (1990), p.312.
14. Vicinus and Nergaard (1990), p.310.
15. McDonald (2001–12), Vol. 14, p.47.
16. Chapple and Pollard (1966), letter 217, p.316.
17. Gaskell (1848), Chapter 16.
18. Gaskell (1866), Chapter 9.
19. Gaskell (1866), Chapter 11.
20. Gaskell (1866), Chapter 19.
21 Gaskell (1866), Chapter 4.
22. Uglow (1993), p.588.
23. Chapple and Pollard (1966), letter 167a, p.250.
24. Gaskell (1866), Chapter 22.
25. Gaskell (1866), Chapter 8.
26. Gaskell (1866), Chapter 17.
27. Gaskell (1866), Chapter 18.
28. Gaskell (1866), Chapter 51.
29. Gaskell (1848), Chapter 8.
30. Gaskell (1866), Chapter 23.
31. Gaskell (1855), Chapter 22.

32. Chapple and Pollard (1966), letter 255, p.358.
33. McDonald (2001–12), Vol. 1, p.83.
34. Gaskell (1848), Chapter 16.

Chapter 10: Where have all the mothers gone?

Where mothers' quotes are not referenced, this is because they come from statements made to me, either in writing or in one of my Mothers Talking discussion meetings.

1. Wakefield, Mary (2023), 'I regret not having more children' (*The Spectator*, 14 October 2023).
2. Barnett (2025), p.79.
3. Lough, Catherine (2023), 'I felt un-feminist to want children, says BBC presenter Alex Jones' (*The Daily Telegraph*, 12 January 2023).
4. Denyer, Lucy (2024), 'Parental stress is at an all-time high' (The *Daily Telegraph*, 30 August 2024, p.7).
5. Hinsliff, Gaby (2015), 'Remaining childless can be wise and meaningful. The pope should know.' (*The Guardian*, 13 February 2015).
6. Unsigned column (2024), 'Having a baby is wonderful, but it isn't the root of female empowerment' (*The Sunday Telegraph*, 7 April 2024, p.7).
7. Wilkinson, Abi (2003), 'Hunt can't nag mothers back to work' (*The Guardian*, 20 February 2003).
8. Jones (2023), p.134.
9. Jones (2023), p.267.
10. Ennis (2014), p.30. Brown was one of several researchers to test whether mothers believed there were 'Mommy Wars' between 'working' and 'stay-at-home' mothers, and to conclude that their data did not confirm the existence of 'Mommy Wars'. See Brown, Solveig 'It's time to move beyond the "Mommy Wars"', also Janacek Reeber, Brianne and Caplan, Paula J. 'Are "Mommy Wars" real?' both in Reid Boyd and Letherby (2014).
11. Reid Boyd and Letherby (2014), pp.289-290.
12. Shore (2006), p.15.
13. For example, see Temkin (1956), pp.88-89. Soranus of Ephesus was a highly reputed ancient Greek physician who lived during the first and second centuries AD.
14. Fildes, Valerie (1979), 'It's a wonder babies ever survived' (*Nursing Mirror Supplement*, 12 July 1979).
15. Waring (1999), p.xxxix.
16. Kitzinger (1967)
17. Kitzinger (2015), p.235.
18. Kitzinger (1986), p.1.
19. Kitzinger (1986), p.20.
20. Kitzinger (1967), p.219.
21. Balaskas (2023), p.11.

22. Balaskas (2023), p.37.
23. Wiessinger, West and Pitman for La Leche League International (2010). There is now a new edition, *The Art of Breastfeeding*.
24. Gentleman, Amelia (2024), 'I have £7 in my bank account' (*The Guardian*, 25 September 2024, p.4).
25. Nightingale (1979), p.52.
26. McDonald (2001–12), Vol. 2, pp.167-213.
27. The Bible. Isaiah 52:1

Index

EG = Elizabeth Gaskell FN = Florence Nightingale Page numbers of the format e.g. 38 (*191n24*) refer to endnotes. The first number is the page where the reference is found in the text, the number in the brackets indicate the notes page and note number.

Also by Naomi Stadlen

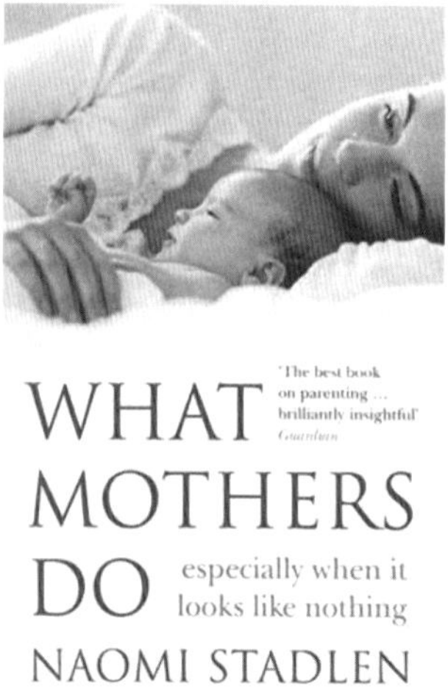

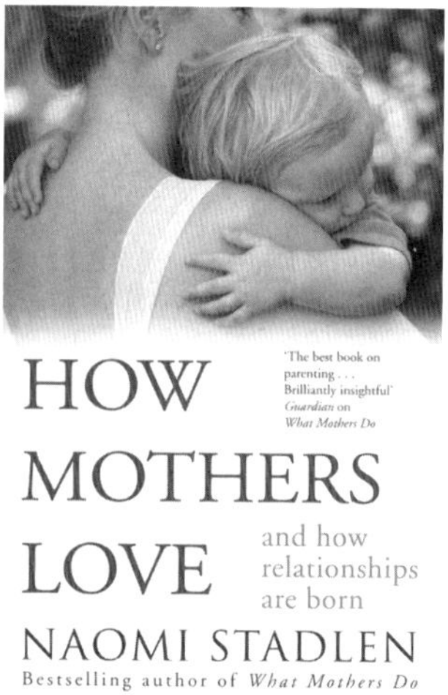

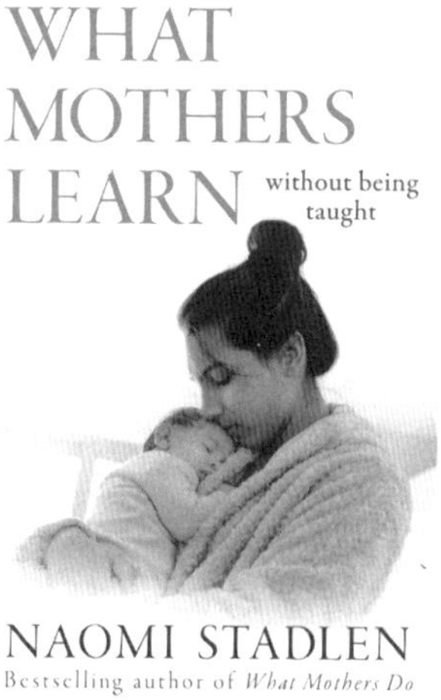

naomistadlen.com